THE
BODY–SMART SYSTEM
The Complete Guide To Cleansing
And Rejuvenation

THE
BODY–SMART
SYSTEM

The Complete Guide To Cleansing And Rejuvenation

Helene Silver

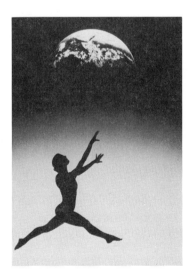

NOTE

This book contains instructions concerning the use of diet, nutritional supplements, herbs and essential oils, and holistic health techniques within the context of a three-week program. However, not all products and techniques should be used by all individuals. This program is not for pregnant women because the dietary restrictions do not provide adequate nutrition for a growing fetus, nor are the herbs and essential oils tested for possible birth defects. This book is not intended as a substitute for the medical advice of a physician. The reader should consult with a physician before embarking on this or any other health program.

For information address: Healthy Healing Publications, 16060 Via Este, Sonora, CA 95370

First Edition by Bantam Books, 1990
©1990 by Helene Silver
ISBN 0-553-05777-4

ISBN 1-884334-60-1

Dedicated to the loving memory of my father,
Sam Silver, whose persistent health problems stimulated
my interest in natural health principles and cures

ACKNOWLEDGMENTS

I gratefully acknowledge my teachers, Walt and Magana Baptiste, pioneers in the natural health movement, for their loving guidance. Many phases of the nutritional, breathing, and yoga portions of the The Body–Smart System, I developed from their teachings. The holistic health philosophers and teachers Edgar Cayce, Dr. Norman Walker, Dr. Bernard Jenson, Dr. Paavo Airola, Dr. Randolph Stone, and Ann Wigmore were all sources of inspiration and information for me over the years.

Special thanks to Kathleen Anderson Ross who did a beautiful job of testing, refining, and quantifying my Body-Smart System recipes.

I express my appreciation to Dr. Elson Haas for his support and medical advice throughout the many years of our association and friendship.

Love and thanks to my close friends and family, especially Gail Schwartz, Trudie London, Joanne Brown, Evelyn Bruenn, Merrily Milmoe, Weslyn Hants, Tim McAteer, Cheryl Silver and Shirley Silver, for nurturing me when I needed it most.

Admiration and gratitude to all of my loyal clients and readers whose trust, discipline, and commitment have taught me so much.

Many thanks to Kathleen Goss and Esther Mitgang for their innumerable contributions to my first edition. An extra special thanks to Rita Aero for her creative contributions to both the first and second editions and for her unflagging confidence in me and the principles I teach.

Much appreciation and gratitude to Kathryn Danielle for her design of this second edition of The Body–Smart System.

Finally, I want to thank Linda Rector Page and Elliot Page of Healthy Healing Publications for their commitment to me and The Body-Smart System over the years. I value our association and shared convictions.

CONTENTS

FOREWORD

by Elson Haas, M.D.

The most simple way I have found to describe symptoms and disease integrates Western thinking, Chinese medicine, and the naturopathic approach to health and illness. Problems in the body and mind often arise from either **deficiencies** or **congestion**. In a state of deficiency, we are not acquiring enough nutrients to meet our bodily needs; whereas, in a state of congestion we are suffering from excessive intake and reduced eliminative functions from the overconsumption of foods and non-foods, such as caffeine, alcohol, nicotine, refined sugar and chemicals.

Those who are deficient may experience symptoms such as fatigue, coldness, hair loss, or dry skin. They need to be nourished with wholesome foods to aid the healing process. Congestive problems, however, are more common in Western, industrialized civilizations. Many of our acute and chronic medical diseases and dilemmas result from the clogging of our tissues and tubes and from the suffocating of our cells and, consequently, of our vitality.

Colds, flus, cancer, cardiovascular diseases, arthritis and allergies are all examples of congestive disorders. These medical problems may be prevented or treated, at least in part and often quite dramatically, by a program of cleansing and detoxification. The incorporation of dietary changes such as those presented in THE BODY–SMART SYSTEM–consumption of more fresh fruits, vegetables and water, and the reduction of animal fats, heavy proteins and abusive substances–is the beginning of the rejuvenation process for the human body. This was discovered long ago and is still true today, although conventional medical science may make light of it in deference to the "quick solution."

I consider the cleansing and detoxification process to be the missing link in Western nutrition and a key to the health and vitality of our civilization. In my two decades of medical practice, I have extensively utilized various cleansing and rejuvenation practices for both myself and literally thousands of patients. I truly believe that these practices are some of the most powerful healing therapies I have seen. They initiate a true healing of ailments rather than simply a suppression of symptoms.

I have written extensively about detoxification in my 1100–page STAYING HEALTHY WITH NUTRITION, where I discuss both the medical and health factors of this important process. However, you have in your hands a beautiful and powerful book, THE BODY–SMART SYSTEM, that can help guide you along your path of healing towards the attainment and maintenance of optimum health.

I have known Helene Silver for nearly 20 years. She is a knowledgeable and devoted practitioner and educator towards the achievement of both inner and outer beauty. In truth, both Helene and I are encouraging you, through our private practices and writing, to take back the responsibility of your health. So much of it is really up to you. It matters how you live–what you do, what you eat, how you think, how you feel. Take hold and do what you can to be vital and healthy. It is really worth it!

Be Well,
Elson M. Haas, M.D.

Dr. Elson M. Haas is a practicing physician of Integrated Medicine and Medical Director of the Preventive Medical Centers of Marin and Sonoma in San Rafael and Cotati, California. Dr. Haas is also the author of the classic preventive medicine text *Staying Healthy With the Seasons* (1981, now in its 20th printing), *Staying Healthy With Nutrition* (1993), and soon to be published *A Diet For All Seasons*. His books are published by Celestial Arts.

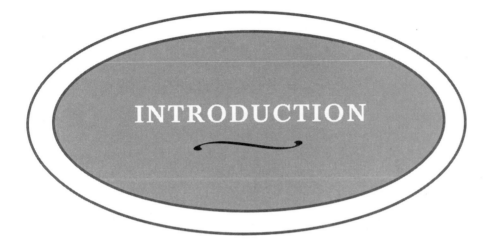

INTRODUCTION

*M*y Cleansing and Rejuvenation Program can change your life. I know, because I have supervised hundreds of clients on a deep–cleansing program like this one. Over and over again, I have watched the pounds and the signs of aging simply melt away, to be replaced by a clarity and optimism that enable people to realize their full potential.

For the past fourteen years, I have been director of the Inner Beauty Institute in Sausalito, California. My clients are well–informed, active adults ranging in age from twenty to sixty–people seeking the most effective, up–to–date methods to maintain their youthful vitality. Whether they find me on their own, or are referred by physicians, chiropractors, massage therapists, or skin care specialists, they all want to experience the benefits of peak health that come from inner cleansing. I place my clients on individualized programs that address their specific concerns–excess weight, constipation, abdominal gas and bloating, skin problems, low energy, premature aging. As they cleanse their bodies of toxins, they enjoy a dramatic rejuvenation of body and mind.

I have been studying the various philosophies and techniques presented in The Body–Smart System for over twenty years and have adapted them for your use. Many of these techniques have been utilized by various cultures for centuries. For the first time, they have been put together in this easy–to–use, comprehensive guide.

I have personally experienced and refined many of these advanced health and beauty techniques and feel better now at forty–seven that I did at thirty! I used to have painful cramping and breast discomfort with my menstrual periods. Thanks to my cleansing and nutritional programs, I no longer have problems with my periods. My skin used to break out all the time; now I receive frequent compliments on my complexion. Ending my old pattern of constipation increased my mental clarity and released a flow of energy that allows me to get through my busy days with enthusiasm and pleasure.

In the past, comprehensive rejuvenation and cleansing programs were available only in expensive spas, where people could retreat to a peaceful, restricted environment, away from the pressures and temptations of their daily lives. Now, using techniques adapted from my Inner Beauty Institute program, you can create a luxurious spa for yourself, in the comfort and privacy of your own home. I will show you how to turn many of your normal daily activities into enjoyable healing rituals. At the end of three short weeks, you will look and feel younger, more attractive, mentally clearer and energized. And you will realize that you can continue to feel this way throughout your life, because you have learned new ways to renew your beauty from the inside out.

My 21-Day Program fine-tunes all the systems of elimination—your skin, your lungs, your lymphatic system, your liver and kidneys, and your colon. Some cleansing methods, such as bathing and skin brushing, may already by familiar to you. Some may be completely new, such as breathing exercises, fasting and colonic irrigations. Through these techniques, you will learn how to release the toxic substances that are clogging up your body and robbing you of youthful beauty and vitality.

You will find that many of these invigorating techniques, activities and special recipes will become favorites that you will integrate into your daily life. Thus, the Program will last much longer than 21 days, and you will use The Body-Smart System as a resource guide for many years to come.

Your most important tool in this cleansing process is clean, pure water. Your body is about 70 percent water. You depend on water to maintain your body temperature, to carry away wastes and toxins, and to renew your body's cells, tissues and fluids. In your at-home spa, you will learn to gently suffuse every part of your body with the miraculous rejuvenative power of water, through bathing, special drinks, and flushes.

To aid in cleansing and detoxifying your body, you will explore the principles of food combining to provide maximum nutrition to every cell in your body, making you more youthful on the outside and healthier inside. You will discover a safe and comfortable approach to fasting. You will learn to stimulate the cleansing action of your lymph system through massage and exercise. You will clear your mind of stressful thoughts by learning how to relax, let go, and return naturally to a positive attitude.

And perhaps most important, at the end of the 21-Day Program you will have learned how to guarantee that the new cells you build will be perfect and healthy because they are free of DNA-damaging toxins.

It takes about three weeks to develop a new habit, and my 21-Day Program is designed to instill new health and beauty habits that you will carry forward into the rest of your life. A convenient weekly shopping list will help

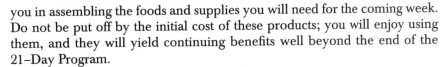

you in assembling the foods and supplies you will need for the coming week. Do not be put off by the initial cost of these products; you will enjoy using them, and they will yield continuing benefits well beyond the end of the 21–Day Program.

You can follow this richly rewarding, intensive program while you continue to go to work and attend to your personal life. Each day's special activities require no more than about sixty minutes. It's an investment of time and pleasurable effort with a big health and beauty payoff. The program worked for me. It works for my clients. And it will work for you!

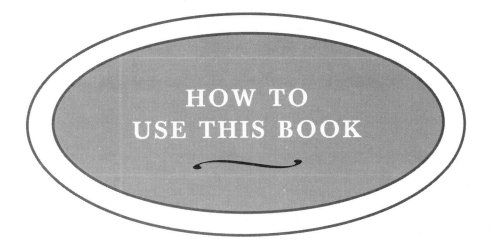

HOW TO
USE THIS BOOK

*T*he Body–Smart System is truly a complete guide to cleansing and rejuvenation!

I will show you how your daily activities such as bathing, breathing, walking, eating, sleeping, eliminating, and thinking can be used to improve your health and appearance. I will give you easy–to–understand and easy–to–follow directions for cleansing your system and developing new healthful, self–nourishing habits.

You will learn how to more effectively use you own "body filters" for daily cleansing of toxins. The improvement will be almost immediate: puffiness under your eyes will disappear, your sleeping and digestion will improve, and your energy will increase!

The rich and famous go to expensive spas regularly to rid themselves of toxins. They know that true beauty is from the inside out, and they can afford to get the best advice and attention available. It works; they usually look quite good! You do not have to leave town to be rejuvenated. You will learn many of the techniques from these sophisticated, international programs simply by reading The Body–Smart System and, whenever you wish, by turning your own home into a "spa."

You may choose to follow the 21–Day Program in its entirety, or you may use the book as a resource and discover recipes, activities and ideas to integrate into and enrich your daily life. I have organized this book with these various uses in mind, so that you will find several "user–friendly" ways for you to proceed.

Perhaps you already know that you want to follow my 21–Day Cleansing and Rejuvenation Program. If so, please begin by reading the Body–Smart Experience on page 7 to familiarize yourself with the content and basic premise of the program. Look over the Body–Smart Schedule beginning on page 37 to familiarize yourself with the program you will be following. At your leisure, read over Chapters 7 through 19 to understand the philosophy behind the program. Then, answer the Self–Assessment Questionnaire beginning on page 14. After doing the questionnaire, proceed with the Goal Setting portion of the program beginning on page 25 to realistically evaluate where you want to go! Finally, read Creating Your Environment beginning on page 31 to prepare the aspects of your everyday life for the program. You will then be ready to begin the 21 days that will change your life!

Perhaps you are not yet ready to follow the 21–Day Cleansing and Rejuvenation Program, but you want to know more about the various systems, techniques and activities that are the very foundation of the Body–Smart Program. Essentially, you may wish to utilize this book as a resource guide to enrich your life. If so, please begin by reading the Body–Smart Experience on page 7 in order to introduce yourself to the basic premise of the program. Jump right into the Self–Assessment Questionnaire on page 14 so that you can understand more fully just which techniques and concepts you want to concentrate on. Finally, at your leisure, read Chapters 7 through 19. I am sure that you will discover many new ideas and begin to integrate your favorite recipes and activities into your daily life. When you feel ready, you can follow the 21–Day Program, or perhaps try one of the shorter programs in Body–Smart Tune–Ups, beginning on page 223.

Regardless of how you use the book, I am certain you will find it a valuable resource for many years to come! You will have more knowledge about how your body works and be able to make more informed, responsible choices as you care for yourself. Over the years, I have done many variations of this program many different times. It always works! You will discover your own individual path through the Body–Smart System–scheduling, meal plans, and activities. That is absolutely fine, and I know that you will be pleased with the results.

As an expert with twenty years in the field of health education, I have discovered many high quality products which promote the goals of cleansing and rejuvenation. These products are discussed throughout the book and can be found in your local health–food store. For your convenience, I have also made them available by mail–order through the Body-Smart Catalog. Please consult the Source Guide on page 231 for ordering information.

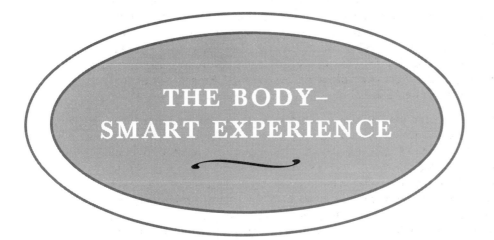

THE BODY-SMART EXPERIENCE

My 21–Day Program is designed to promote a positive, overall change in your lifestyle. While you will undoubtedly lose weight on this program, you will also learn health habits that will stay with you over your lifetime, improving the quality of your life. Your body will last you many youthful–looking years longer, you will be able to give more of yourself to others, and you will experience a greater, more satisfying sense of well–being.

If you are like most of my clients, you want to look and feel the very best you can. You may have decided it is time to lose weight, to clean the toxins out of your body, or to do something about your low energy, poor complexion or constipation.

CLEANSING FOR OPTIMAL HEALTH

Throughout my years of practice as a health educator, I have learned that many health problems are caused by the accumulation of toxic waste in the body. We all know that our bodies require nourishment–food, water, and oxygen. Much emphasis is placed on putting right things into your body, but it is equally important for the waste to leave your body efficiently. The key to maintaining a constant cleansing process in your body is fresh, pure water. Your body is made of more than 70 percent water, and water is an essential component of every cell. When you constantly flush your organs of elimination with water, your body remains clear of waste and is able to make the best possible use of your food and oxygen.

When you consume food, your digestive system breaks it down and utilizes what it needs, and then eliminates the waste, not only through the intestines, but throughout the entire body. You breathe in oxygen through the lungs and exhale waste as carbon dioxide. Your bloodstream and lymph system carry nutrients to the cells and carry away cellular waste. Your skin eliminates waste through sweat and the shedding of dead cells. The water you drink, and which is absorbed from your food, carries away waste products in solution, to be eliminated through the kidneys.

If any of these systems of elimination are clogged up by waste, the whole system begins to back up. Not only does the waste create a toxic condition, but your body is also unable to properly utilize the new nutrients that are put in. If the plumbing in your house were to become plugged up and the garbage collectors were to go on strike, you would no longer be able to dispose of the waste that is produced in the course of the day, and soon your home would be unfit to live in. Your body works in much the same way, and your outer beauty and vitality are affected.

THE HOLISTIC PERSPECTIVE

My cleansing program deals with your body as a whole system. This holistic view is somewhat different from the general medical perspective. Western medicine tends to focus on a specific disease or symptom in a specific part of the body, as if it were isolated from the whole. From the holistic point of view, what goes on in one part of the body is connected to what happens in every other part of the body. The holistic approach looks at what goes on in your mind and your spirit as well as in your body, and recognizes that all these aspects of your being influence and reflect one another.

Rather than looking at health as the absence of disease, the holistic approach defines health in terms of a positive model of wellness. The wellness model goes beyond the absence of symptoms to encourage a high level of functioning on the physical, mental, and spiritual planes. I define wellness as a creative process of growth and change, where we take responsibility for using our bodies, minds, and emotions in a constructive way, and recognize our connection to a larger community of beings. Such self–responsibility and caring are the ultimate goals of my program. I do not promise you any "magic bullet" to eliminate isolated symptoms. Rather, I am offering you a holistic approach, to bring out the very best in your physical functioning, your mind, emotions, and spirit.

FOOD, WATER, AND AIR–THE PRINCIPLES OF THE PROGRAM

You may be wondering how you can incorporate all the activities of an At-Home Program into your busy daily life. The 21–Day Program transforms the activities that you do every day–bathing, breathing, walking, eating, thinking, sleeping–into positive, enjoyable, rejuvenating rituals. We all have spent a great deal of time and money going to diet doctors, having facials, and attending exercise classes and gyms. As you learn the principles of this program, you will be able to provide much of this health and beauty care for yourself at home.

The Clean and Clear Food Philosophy

We begin with food, eliminating the toxins that you are putting into your body needlessly and unintentionally. I encourage you to buy only organically grown fruits and vegetables. Commercially grown produce is treated with a frightening variety of chemicals–pesticides, herbicides, fungicides, bleaches, and gases, among others. Because the body is not designed to metabolize these man–made compounds, many of them are stored as toxic waste. If you are not able to obtain organic fruits and vegetables, I will show you how to cleanse your produce so you will not introduce more toxins into your body.

Because much animal protein today is also contaminated with drugs and chemicals, I will ask you to limit your animal–flesh consumption to organic chicken and deep–water ocean fish such as swordfish, tuna, sea bass, and halibut. I want you to eat whole, fresh foods as often as possible, to furnish your cells and tissues with all the nutrients they require for youthful beauty and vitality. I will show you how to combine foods properly so you will get the greatest possible benefit from them, create the smallest amount of toxic residue, and reduce the strain on your digestive system.

On the Clean and Clear Diet you will be eating delicious, nourishing meals that will leave you feeling rejuvenated and happy. Most people shed five to twenty pounds during the program. My program also allows for individual variation. For example, some people simply do not do well on a light breakfast of fruit alone. Please pay attention to your body's messages and plan for the suggested midmorning protein drink if your energy level has a tendency to drop before lunchtime, or if you tend to have an appetite in the morning. Similarly, if you really feel better having your protein meal in the evening, you are free to adjust your menus accordingly, as long as you continue to adhere to the rules of food combining you will be learning in this program. Those of you who choose not to eat animal products will also find it easy and convenient to follow the principles of the Clean and Clear Diet.

The Water Prescription

Just as important as your food is the water you drink. Every cell in your body is constantly flushed and bathed by an exchange of water that brings in nutrients to build new cells and carries away waste. Pure, clean water is a very important element of your daily intake. The quality of tap water in the United States varies widely from place to place. More than seven hundred toxic compounds have been identified in water drawn from U.S. water systems. Even if your municipal water supply is free of bacteria, it may contain high levels of chlorine and rust, which, combined with other substances, can form unhealthy compounds.

The best health protection today is to use purified water. Many people drink bottled water–which may be distilled, filtered spring water, or well water–because they distrust the water from their tap. Unfortunately, water bottling is an essentially unregulated industry. One bottled–water company was found to be selling municipal tap water that had been labeled spring water. Another company was getting its water from a well adjacent to a toxic dump site. If you are not confident about the purity of the bottled water available to you, I recommend that you install a water purifier on your tap.

It is very easy to do. The water purifier that I prefer uses an activated charcoal–block filter, which is capable of removing organic chemicals, bacteria, chlorine, toxic metals, dirt, and other suspended matter, while leaving the beneficial natural minerals dissolved in the water. In some areas, where the water is very contaminated, it may be necessary to use a reverse osmosis filter, which removes contaminants by means of a semipermeable membrane, in combination with a charcoal–block filter. Whichever you choose, I recommend that you change the filter in your water purifier twice as often as recommended by the manufacturer.

In any case, use nothing but purified water during your 21–Day Program for making all your teas, beverages, soups, and recipes, as well as for your daily drinking water. If you must resort to bottled water, do not use carbonated water, because it just adds gas and bloating to your system. You should also be suspicious of European bottled waters since the Chernobyl incident, because they may contain radioactive particles.

Besides the water you drink, you will be exploring the external uses of water for healing and rejuvenation. Your daily showers and baths will be one of the most enjoyable aspects of this program. Bathing is an essential practice in all the world's great health spas. To enrich your bathing rituals and make them even more pleasurable, I will show you how to use aromatic essential oils to relax your body and your mind and to produce specific healing and beautifying effects. They also create wonderful scents in your bath.

Essential Breathing

I will help you to become aware of your breathing, and to use it to cleanse your body and free your mind of stress. Stress reduction is one of the most important parts of any rejuvenation program. I will show you many techniques for becoming more aware of where you are holding stress in your body, and releasing that stress. I will encourage you to get plenty of rest, using bathing and stress–releasing evening activities to ease yourself into sleep. The quality of your sleep reflects the quality of your waking state. By learning to have a more relaxed, vital and joyful daytime life, you will also enjoy a more pleasant, restful, and beneficial sleep. Finally, as you clean out your body, I will also encourage you to clear your mind of negative thoughts, and to use your thinking in a positive constructive way.

Populations renowned for their longevity and vitality have much to teach us about how to eat right, relieve stress, and maintain an active lifestyle and a positive mental attitude. My 21–Day Program includes proven health, beauty, and rejuvenation secrets from around the world–foods such as sea vegetables, garlic, onions, and fermented foods, and healing practices such as bathing and massage. In addition, my program brings you the very latest discoveries in nutrition and life–extension research, introducing you to supplements and skin–care products that promise to be the most exciting new beauty and health–care products of the decade.

THE THREE WEEKS OF THE PROGRAM

The At–Home Program consists of three weeks of scheduled activities. Before beginning the program, I suggest that you read Chapters 7 through

19 in order to introduce yourself to important components of the program—diet, exercise, skin care, bathing, breathing, and massage.

The First Week

The 21–Day Program has three phases. During the first, or elimination phase, you will begin to clean out your body by eliminating sources of toxins in your diet, concentrating on whole, organic foods and clean, pure water. You will take a look at your habits, and eliminate sources of toxicity. At the same time, you will gradually develop positive new habits, as you learn how to make the best possible use of exercise, breathing, bathing, and massage to promote cleansing, rejuvenation, beauty, and a feeling of vitality.

The Second Week

During the cleansing phase, you will be clearing your body of wastes more intensely, because you will be eliminating animal protein from your diet and consuming an array of fruits and vegetables, and finally only juices and broth for two days. By this time, you will have eliminated many of the foods to which people are often unknowingly sensitive. You may experience some minor symptoms, such as a light headache or a pimple or two, as your body begins to throw off the toxins that are being released from the cells. You will also practice techniques for colon cleansing, and your body will become progressively cleaner, clearer, and lighter. You will discover that the cleansing process is not only physical but also psychological. Often, as people clean out their bodies, they find that they are also releasing long–held emotions; they may also experience profound personal insights during this time. In working with my clients, I have been amazed to see how the cleansing process brings the mind and body into greater harmony.

The Third Week

As you return to a normal diet during the third, or reintroduction, phase, you will practice techniques to conquer constipation and eliminate cellulite forever. Did you know that laxatives are the best selling over–the–counter remedy in this country? Many people reading this book have probably suffered from constipation or poor elimination habits, and may be seeking help for this problem. Constipation results in the buildup of toxic–waste material in your colon—wastes that are periodically absorbed into your body, aging it. I am going to help you get rid of this toxic waste, and show you how to prevent it from building up in the future. This toxic waste is also a major factor in the formation of cellulite—those unattractive, lumpy deposits of fat, water, and waste that ruin many otherwise good figures. By showing you how to avoid constipation forever, I will also help you to keep cellulite from forming in your body. In addition, my cleansing program, along with special cellulite–reducing activities, will help you to reduce any cellulite you may now have.

Truly, by learning to respect, love and take responsibility for your body, you are also assisting the entire planet. By clearing out the pollution in your body, you become more aware of the commitment needed to purify and heal our fragile, shared environment.

NOTES TO MYSELF

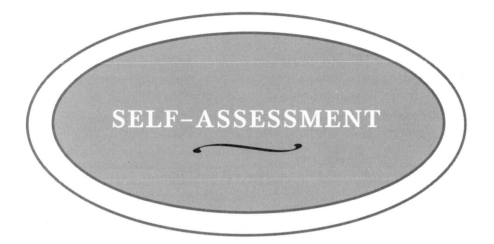

SELF–ASSESSMENT

*N*ow that you understand the basic principles of my Cleansing and Rejuvenation Program, let's decide if it's for you by examining where you are right now.

I always begin my first appointment with clients by helping them to examine their health and set realistic goals. I help them to evaluate every aspect of their lives—diet, exercise, stress tolerance, relationships, the environment they live in. I have adapted my client questionnaire so that you can go through this process on your own. In filling out this questionnaire, try to be totally honest with yourself. Sometimes it takes my clients weeks or months before they feel comfortable telling me certain things; but you can start out with a completely honest inventory of your own health practices and concerns. You may become aware of some aspects of your life that you never thought of as contributing to how you look and feel.

After you have filled out and scored the questionnaire, make time to take a walk for a least thirty minutes. On an unconscious level, what you have learned about yourself in the questionnaire will be sinking in. Try not to think as you walk! Find a place close to nature where you can walk, even if you must drive or take a bus there. Open yourself up to your surroundings. Pay attention to your breathing, and allow yourself to be refreshed by the sights, sounds, and smells of the outdoors.

When you return, you will be ready to set goals for what you hope to accomplish in your 21–Day Program. Or, perhaps you have decided to do the program at another time. If so, you will skip over the chapter on Setting Your Goals and begin to read Chapters 8 through 20. In either case, you will have a clearer picture of your level of health and your commitment to yourself.

ORIENTATION QUESTIONNAIRE

In order to make changes in how you look and feel, it will be helpful to evaluate your present health practices and level of awareness. This questionnaire will help you to identify areas you may want to work on during the 21–Day Program.

Instructions

For each question, answer Y for yes or often, S for sometimes or somewhat, and N for no or rarely. After you have completed the questionnaire, refer to the Scoring Key to determine your score on each section. In the next chapter I will tell you how to use your scores for goal-setting.

		Y	S	N
1.	**DIET**			
a.	Do you make a point of eating natural, whole foods?	☐	☐	☐
b.	Do you eat animal protein more than once a day?	☐	☐	☐
c.	Do you eat packaged or processed foods?	☐	☐	☐
d.	Do you make an effort to avoid insecticides and other chemicals in foods	☐	☐	☐
e.	Do you ever notice any physical or mental symptoms (e.g. headache, stomach pain, rash, drowsiness, irritability) after eating a certain food?	☐	☐	☐
f.	Do you eat fresh fruits or vegetables every day?	☐	☐	☐
g.	Do you drink six to eight glasses of water every day?	☐	☐	☐
h.	Do you drink tap water?	☐	☐	☐
2.	**EATING HABITS**			
a.	Do you eat in a calm, relaxed setting, without distractions?	☐	☐	☐
b.	If you are angry or upset, do you try to calm down before eating?	☐	☐	☐
c.	Do you chew your food well?	☐	☐	☐
d.	Do you tend to overeat?	☐	☐	☐
e.	Do you eat when you are not hungry?	☐	☐	☐
f.	Do you regularly eat out in restaurants?	☐	☐	☐

3. WEIGHT CONTROL   Y   S   N

a. Are you comfortable with your present weight?   ☐   ☐   ☐

b. Are you overweight?   ☐   ☐   ☐

c. Are you underweight?   ☐   ☐   ☐

d. Do you have a history of crash dieting?   ☐   ☐   ☐

e. Do you tend to eat compulsively to avoid dealing with   ☐   ☐   ☐
   emotional issues?

4. DIGESTION

a. Do you often feel bloated and full after eating?   ☐   ☐   ☐

b. Do you notice after eating particular foods that you   ☐   ☐   ☐
   tend to be bloated or uncomfortable?

c. Do you experience heartburn or gas pains after eating?   ☐   ☐   ☐

5. ELIMINATION

a. Do you move your bowels every day?   ☐   ☐   ☐

b. Do you move your bowels in direct proportion to what   ☐   ☐   ☐
   you eat (i.e. two meals a day equals two bowel
   movements?)

c. Are your stools hard?   ☐   ☐   ☐

d. Are you generally constipated?   ☐   ☐   ☐

e. Do you get constipated before your menstrual period?   ☐   ☐   ☐

6. ENERGY LEVEL

a. Would you describe your energy level as generally   ☐   ☐   ☐
   low?

b. Are you aware of the fluctuations in your energy level   ☐   ☐   ☐
   during the day?

c. Are these changes in energy level so dramatic that   ☐   ☐   ☐
   they keep you from doing things you would like to do?

d. Does your energy level seem to increase or decrease in   ☐   ☐   ☐
   relation to meals?

		Y	S	N

e. As you grow older, do you notice your energy level decreasing? ☐ ☐ ☐

7. EXERCISE

a. Would you describe yourself as physically fit? ☐ ☐ ☐

b. Do you do some form of aerobic activity, such as brisk walking, for one-half hour at least three times a week? ☐ ☐ ☐

c. Do you do yoga or other stretching exercises? ☐ ☐ ☐

d. Do you walk or ride a bicycle regularly, rather than taking a bus or car? ☐ ☐ ☐

8. BREATHING

a. Do you have frequent respiratory infections or bronchitis? ☐ ☐ ☐

b. Does your abdomen expand when you breathe? ☐ ☐ ☐

c. Do you tend to breathe through your mouth? ☐ ☐ ☐

d. Do you do any regular breathing exercises? ☐ ☐ ☐

e. Do you notice that you hold your breath or hyperventilate when you are nervous or angry? ☐ ☐ ☐

9. REST AND SLEEP

a. Do you sleep six to eight hours a night? ☐ ☐ ☐

b. Do you sleep more than nine hours at night? ☐ ☐ ☐

c. Do you have trouble falling asleep? ☐ ☐ ☐

d. Do you have trouble getting up in the morning? ☐ ☐ ☐

e. Do you wake up during the night? ☐ ☐ ☐

10. STRESS LEVEL

a. Would you rate the general stress level in your life as high? ☐ ☐ ☐

b. Do you hold a lot of stress in your body? ☐ ☐ ☐

		Y	S	N

c. Do you know which parts of your body tend to become tense or painful when you are under stress? ☐ ☐ ☐

d. Does your job produce stress for you? ☐ ☐ ☐

e. Do your family or your personal relationships produce stress for you? ☐ ☐ ☐

f. Are you able to express your anger? ☐ ☐ ☐

11. GENERAL APPEARANCE AND PERSONAL HYGIENE

a. Do you feel that you are too rapidly showing signs of aging? ☐ ☐ ☐

b. Do you floss your teeth every day? ☐ ☐ ☐

c. Are your teeth in need of repair? ☐ ☐ ☐

d. Do you have bad breath? ☐ ☐ ☐

e. Do you have an unpleasant body odor? ☐ ☐ ☐

f. Do you look bloated or puffy? ☐ ☐ ☐

g. Do you have a protruding tummy, in spite of all your efforts at diet and exercise? ☐ ☐ ☐

12. SKIN, HAIR, AND NAILS

a. Is your skin either extremely dry or very oily? ☐ ☐ ☐

b. Do you often have blemishes on your face, back, or other parts of the body? ☐ ☐ ☐

c. Is your hair dry and dull? ☐ ☐ ☐

d. Are your nails weak, ridged, or bitten? ☐ ☐ ☐

e. Do you have cellulite? ☐ ☐ ☐

f. Do you use antiperspirants or deodorants containing aluminum or other chemical compounds? ☐ ☐ ☐

13. MENSTRUAL CYCLE

a. Does your menstrual period occur in a regular cycle? ☐ ☐ ☐

b. Is the flow about the same every cycle? ☐ ☐ ☐

	Y	S	N
c. Do you have severe menstrual cramps?	☐	☐	☐
d. Do you have a lot of bloating before your period?	☐	☐	☐
e. Do you have an increased tendency to get angry, anxious, or depressed just before your period?	☐	☐	☐
f. Are you having any uncomfortable symptoms as a result of nearing or undergoing menopause?	☐	☐	☐

14. SEXUALITY

	Y	S	N
a. Are you satisfied with your sexual drive?	☐	☐	☐
b. Does decreased or excessive libido cause problems in your relationship?	☐	☐	☐
c. Do you crave more touch or nurturing than you are presently receiving?	☐	☐	☐
d. Do you practice "safe sex"?	☐	☐	☐

15. EMOTIONAL AND MENTAL HEALTH

	Y	S	N
a. Do you notice mood swings throughout the day, the week, or the month?	☐	☐	☐
b. Do you get angry easily?	☐	☐	☐
c. Do you cry easily?	☐	☐	☐
d. Do you laugh a lot?	☐	☐	☐
e. Do you use any stimulants, depressants, or other drugs (legal or illegal) to affect your mood or alertness?	☐	☐	☐

16. SUBSTANCE USE

	Y	S	N
a. Do you drink more than one caffeine beverage each day?	☐	☐	☐
b. Are you concerned about your tobacco use?	☐	☐	☐
c. Do you drink alcohol more than you think you should?	☐	☐	☐
d. Do you need support in dealing with your use of any of these substances?	☐	☐	☐

	Y	S	N

17. ENVIRONMENT

a. Are you pleased with the overall appearance and atmosphere of your home environment? ☐ ☐ ☐

b. Do you have natural light, fresh air, and green plants or access to nature in your living space? ☐ ☐ ☐

c. Is there a quiet place in your home where you can have complete privacy for an hour or more? ☐ ☐ ☐

Questionnaire Scoring Key

Use the following key to score your responses on the Orientation Questionnaire. Circle your answers, and total the scores for each section. Record them in the box provided. If your score for a given section is equal to or higher than the Goal Trigger Score, this may indicate an area of special concern.

1. DIET

	Y	S	N
a	0	1	2
b	2	1	0
c	2	1	0
d	0	1	2
e	2	1	0
f	0	1	2
g	0	1	2
h	2	1	0	TOTAL

Goal Trigger Score: 7

2. EATING HABITS

	Y	S	N
a	0	1	2
b	0	1	2
c	0	1	0
d	2	1	0
e	2	1	0
f	2	1	0	TOTAL

Goal Trigger Score: 5

3. WEIGHT CONTROL

	Y	S	N
a	0	1	2
b	2	1	0
c	2	1	0
d	2	1	0
e	2	1	0	TOTAL

Goal Trigger Score: 4

4. DIGESTION

	Y	S	N
a	2	1	0
b	2	1	0
c	2	1	0	TOTAL

Goal Trigger Score: 4

5. ELIMINATION

	Y	S	N
a	1	2	4
b	1	1	2
c	2	1	0
d	2	1	0
e	2	1	0	TOTAL

Goal Trigger Score: 5

6. ENERGY LEVEL

	Y	S	N
a	2	1	0
b	0	1	2
c	2	1	0
d	2	1	0
e	2	1	0	TOTAL

Goal Trigger Score: 6

7. EXERCISE

	Y	S	N
a	0	2	4
b	0	1	2
c	0	1	2
d	0	1	2	TOTAL

Goal Trigger Score: 4

8. BREATHING

	Y	S	N
a	2	1	0
b	0	1	2
c	2	1	0
d	0	1	2
e	2	1	0	TOTAL

Goal Trigger Score: 4

9. REST AND SLEEP

	Y	S	N	
a	0	1	2	
b	2	1	0	
c	4	2	0	
d	2	1	0	
e	2	1	0	TOTAL

Goal Trigger Score: 6

10. STRESS LEVEL

	Y	S	N	
a	4	2	0	
b	2	1	0	
c	0	1	2	
d	2	1	0	
e	2	1	0	
f	0	1	2	TOTAL

Goal Trigger Score: 6

11. GENERAL APPEARANCE AND PERSONAL HYGIENE

	Y	S	N	
a	4	2	0	
b	0	1	2	
c	2	1	0	
d	2	1	0	
e	2	1	0	
f	2	1	0	
g	2	1	0	TOTAL

Goal Trigger Score: 8

12. SKIN, HAIR AND NAILS

	Y	S	N	
a	2	1	0	
b	2	1	0	
c	2	1	0	
d	2	1	0	
e	2	1	0	
f	2	1	0	TOTAL

Goal Trigger Score: 6

13. MENSTRUAL CYCLE

	Y	S	N	
a	0	1	2	
b	0	1	2	
c	2	1	0	
d	2	1	0	
e	2	1	0	
f	4	2	0	TOTAL

Goal Trigger Score: 6

14. SEXUALITY

	Y	S	N	
a	0	1	2	
b	2	1	0	
c	2	1	0	
d	0	2	4	TOTAL

Goal Trigger Score: 4

15. EMOTIONAL AND MENTAL HEALTH

	Y	S	N	
a	2	1	0	
b	2	1	0	
c	2	1	0	
d	0	1	2	
e	2	1	0	TOTAL

Goal Trigger Score: 5

16. SUBSTANCE USE

	Y	S	N	
a	2	1	0	
b	2	1	0	
c	2	1	0	
d	4	2	0	TOTAL

Goal Trigger Score: 6

17. ENVIRONMENT

	Y	S	N	
a	0	2	4	
b	0	1	2	
c	0	1	2	TOTAL

Goal Trigger Score: 4

Circle the boxes where your totals are equal to or higher than the Goal Trigger Score. Keep these areas in mind as you decide your course of action regarding the Cleansing and Rejuvenation Program.

TOXICITY SYMPTOM CHECKLIST

Many different conditions can be indications of toxicity in the system. Before beginning the 21–Day Program, complete the Toxicity Symptom Checklist to evaluate your present toxicity level. Put today's date at the top of the first column, and then score yourself for each of the symptoms listed according to the following scale:

> 0 = absent
>
> 1 = mild
>
> 2 = moderate
>
> 3 = severe

Add up your scores for today's date, for a total toxicity score. After you have finished the 21–Day Program, you will notice a marked drop in your toxicity level. Retest yourself at the end of this program (on Day 21), again three months later (on Day 21 + 90 days), and then at three–month intervals, as you continue to incorporate your new lifestyle practices into your daily routine.

SYMPTOM	(Day 2) DATE:	(Day 21) DATE:	(Day 21 + 90 days) DATE:
	_____	_____	_____
Overweight or underweight	_____	_____	_____
Abdominal pain, tenderness, or cramping	_____	_____	_____
Protruding abdomen	_____	_____	_____
Heartburn	_____	_____	_____
Gas, burping, or flatulence	_____	_____	_____
Bad breath	_____	_____	_____
Coated tongue	_____	_____	_____

Offensive Body Odor   ____   ____   ____

Skin blemishes or sallow
complexion   ____   ____   ____

Dark circles under the eyes   ____   ____   ____

Facial puffiness   ____   ____   ____

Fluid retention or bloating   ____   ____   ____

Dry or brittle hair   ____   ____   ____

Brittle nails   ____   ____   ____

Low back pain   ____   ____   ____

Premenstrual tension   ____   ____   ____

Premenstrual or menstrual
discomfort (e.g. sorebreasts,
bloating)   ____   ____   ____

Sore joints   ____   ____   ____

Reduced sexual desire   ____   ____   ____

Headaches   ____   ____   ____

Fatigue   ____   ____   ____

Depression   ____   ____   ____

Irritability or anxiety   ____   ____   ____

Low energy   ____   ____   ____

TOTAL TOXICITY SCORE: ☐   ☐   ☐

Congratulations! By taking the Self-Assessment Questionnaire and doing the Toxicity Symptom Checklist as honestly as possible, you have taken a big step forward in your commitment to yourself and your level of health. You are preparing to be the very best that you can be. Take some time now to relax and think about whether you would like to proceed with the 21–Day Program. If so, go on to the next chapter so that you can set your personal goals for the program. If you are not ready or you have not decided, that's really OK! You may skip the chapter on Setting Your Goals and read on from Chapters 8 through 20. You can come back to set your goals at any time!

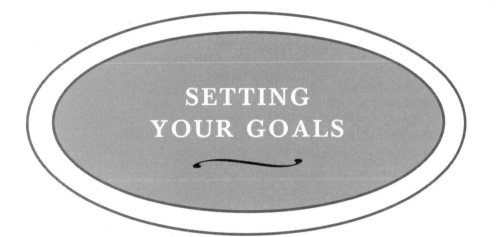

SETTING
YOUR GOALS

When you filled out your questionnaire and scored yourself, you no doubt became aware of things that you would like to focus on during the course of the 21–Day Program. Goal–setting is one of the most crucial parts of your whole program, because it is when you chart the course that you will follow for the entire three weeks.

It is important to establish realistic goals. Do not strive to be perfect, or expect to achieve your goals or make meaningful changes overnight. Part of the benefit of this program is that it is fun, and helps you to feel good about yourself. You may repeat the program several times during the next year, and each time you can set more advanced goals. The key is to be gentle with yourself, and to make this an enjoyable experience.

Try to define your goals in the form of positive statements. For example, instead of saying, "I don't want to have a bloated stomach after meals," you can say, "I want to feel clean and clear and light after meals." Instead of saying, "I don't want to feel angry and tense at work," make your goal, "I want to be calm and good–humored at work." Stating your goals in an affirmative way reinforces your positive self–image.

Do not try to define goals in every area on the questionnaire. I want you to concentrate on setting goals only in those areas of your life that are especially important to you, where your own choices can make a difference. Keep in mind that changing your attitude is just as important as changing your behavior. Feel free to set goals that do not involve spectacular outward changes. As you change yourself within, the external things will improve noticeably.

Go back and review your scores on the Orientation Questionnaire. For each section of the questionnaire, I have provided a Goal Trigger Score. If your score is equal to or higher than this Goal Trigger Score, circle or highlight your score. This is an area where you will probably want to set some goals. Finally, go back over the questionnaire and see if there are any areas that are of special concern to you, even if your score for that section is not high. Mark those sections also.

Now, go to the areas of concern below that have been triggered in the scoring of your questionnaire, or that you have marked as significant for you. Here you will find some suggestions that will help you to state your goals. Record your goals under the corresponding headings in the 21–Day Goals Contract on page 29.

1. Diet Practices. Most of your concerns in this area will be taken care of simply by eating natural, whole foods and eliminating processed foods on the Clean and Clear Diet I will introduce in Chapter 8. If a sweet tooth is an area of special concern, an example of a realistic and positive goal might be, "I will replace my craving for sugar with an enjoyment of fresh fruits."

2. Eating Habits. As I will explain in Chapter 8, The Clean and Clear Diet, your emotional and mental state have a direct bearing on your ability to digest your food. You will learn many ways to calm and center yourself during this program–for example, through relaxing baths on pages 152 through 158, through yoga postures on pages 123 through 131, and through the breathing exercises on pages 135 through 139. A possible goal might be, "I will eat only when I am calm"; or, "I will eat slowly, chew my food well, and pay attention to its flavor, texture, and smell."

3. Weight Control. If you want to lose (or gain) weight, set a realistic goal for yourself. Although your weight will tend to normalize on the 21–Day Program, the main objective is not rapid weight loss, but lifelong dietary change. The Clean and Clear Diet, accompanied by the tips I will offer for lifelong bowel health, will help to keep your weight where you want it to be.

4. Digestion. In Chapter 8, The Clean and Clear Diet, you will learn how your digestive system works and why you may have been having problems with digestive upset in the past. Special cleansing beverages and digestion–toning postures will help to flush and heal your digestive system during Week 2. If digestive problems are one of your reasons for undertaking this program, you may want to set a positive overall goal, such as, "I will learn how to select foods in such a way that I will feel light and comfortable after my meals."

5. Elimination. If you are troubled by constipation, the Clean and Clear Diet will automatically help you to resolve this problem. The cleansing process will become more intense during Weeks 2 and 3 as you flush all your systems of elimination and. practice colon cleansing. You will learn rules for eliminating constipation forever. A realistic goal might be, "I will use natural methods for keeping my bowel function regular."

6. Energy Level. As you eliminate the toxins from your system through proper diet, you will begin to experience an increase in your energy level.

Your exercise program and yoga postures are also designed to improve your energy level, as are the invigorating baths utilized throughout the program. If low or fluctuating energy levels have been limiting your activity or keeping you dependent on caffeine, state a goal such as, "I will become aware of the daily fluctuations in my energy level, and learn natural ways to increase my energy when I need an extra boost."

7. Exercise. In Chapter 10, Movement Into Health, I will introduce a simple, pleasant program of brisk walking that can keep you in shape for the rest of your life. If you have been irregular in your commitment to exercise in the past, a general goal might be, "I will walk whenever possible, for pleasure, exercise, and transportation."

8. Breathing. The essential breathing exercises on pages 135 through 139 and the breath–awareness activities that accompany your daily exercise will improve your breathing capacity. A general goal might be, "I will pay attention to my breathing, and learn how to use breathing exercises for health and relaxation."

9. Rest and Sleep. It is important to get plenty of sleep during the program to support the physical and emotional changes that you will be experiencing. Commit yourself to a certain number of hours of sleep every night. If you suffer from insomnia or early awakening, the 21–Day Program will provide many aids to help solve these problems, such as the relaxing baths on pages 152 through 158 and the various forms of massage described in Chapter 15, Massage and Renew Yourself. A general goal might be, "I will practice natural methods for inducing sleep."

10. Stress Level. Everyone experiences stress. The first step in learning to control stress is to learn to recognize it in your body and your mind. Awareness exercises, such as the tense–and–relax Yoga Stress Releaser on page 124, can help you take a regular inventory of your stress points. You will then be able to use breathing, exercise, bathing, and mental reprogramming—all explained in this program—to control the stress you have identified. A realistic goal might be, "I will learn to recognize the signs of stress in my body, and I will practice techniques to release my daily stress."

11. General Appearance and Personal Hygiene. Even with all the pleasurable bathing activities recommended throughout the 21–Day Program, it is still up to you to maintain high standards of cleanliness and personal care. You may find that the intensive cleansing during Week 2 will help resolve some troublesome problems, such as unpleasant body odor, bad breath, or a protruding tummy. Other issues will require your specific attention and resolve. An example of a realistic goal might be, "I will establish the habit of flossing my teeth every day" or, "I will only use a natural, chemical–free deodorant."

12. Skin, Hair, and Nails. As you follow the Clean and Clear Diet and the skin–care program described in Chapter 12, Beautiful Skin: From the Inside Out, your complexion should become clear and glowing with youthful radiance. Special unsaturated–oil supplements introduced in the diet will help make your hair shiny and your nails healthy and strong. Still, there are some areas where you may need to make personal decisions and commitments. A realistic goal might be, "I will replace my cosmetics and skin–care products with all natural products" or, "I will devote extra effort to the special activities to rid my body of cellulite."

13. Menstrual Cycle. A special chapter "For Women Only" on page 213 will provide helpful suggestions for overcoming menstrual discomfort naturally. The regular exercise program you will establish during the 21–Day Program, as well as reducing your overall toxicity, should also help to keep your cycle normal and regular. A realistic goal might be, "I will become more in tune with my monthly cycle, and use it as an opportunity for cleansing."

14. Sexuality. Some, but by no means all, sexual problems are related to toxicity and stress. The conscious breathing techniques you will learn in Chapter 11, Breathe Your Way to Youth, may prove especially useful in helping you to relax and open yourself sexually. In Chapter 15, Massage and Renew Yourself, you will learn how to use massage to satisfy the normal human need for nurturing, nonsexual touch. You may also be surprised to discover during Week 2 that colon cleansing can produce a dramatic improvement in many people's sex lives. A realistic goal in this area might be, "I will learn new ways to give and receive pleasure and express caring."

15. Emotional and Mental Health. Emotional and mental problems are often the result of toxicity, lack of exercise, or excessive stress. During Week 2, you will undergo an intensive cleansing, accompanied by the use of affirmations to reprogram your negative thinking into positive attitudes. The 21–Day Program provides many natural techniques for feeling good about your whole self. A realistic general goal might be, "I will be more easygoing and cultivate a sense of humor about the little things that bother me," or, "I will spend my time with positive, upbeat, like–minded people."

16. Substance Use. This is an area where you will really need to take a look at what kind of commitment you want to make. I do not insist that you quit drinking coffee, smoking, or drinking alcohol, completely. If you want to eliminate or cut down on any of your toxic habits, set realistic goals for yourself, so you do not waste energy and create stress by blaming yourself for slipping. On page 135 I will give you some ideas about how to cut down on smoking.

17. Environment. In the Questionnaire I have encouraged you to think about your environment. Perhaps you have already begun to think of ways to make your home more peaceful and pleasing. What changes would you like to make in your personal environment? It may not be realistic to set a goal of moving to the country, but you can think of ways to help keep the air in your house clean or to protect yourself from excessive noise. A positive goal might be, "I will create a quiet, private place where I can enjoy being by myself."

Now, fill in your goals on the 21–Day Goals Contract on the next page. Remember, make commitments only in those areas where you have real concerns.

21-Day Goals Contract

During the 21-Day At-Home Program and after its completion, I commit myself to making the following changes:

1. Diet: _____

2. Eating Habits: _____

3. Weight Control: _____

4. Digestion: _____

5. Elimination: _____

6. Energy Level: _____

7. Exercise: _____

8. Breathing: _____

9. Rest and Sleep: _____

10. Stress Level: _____

11. General Appearance and Personal Hygiene: _____

    _____

12. Skin, Hair, and Nails: _____

13. Menstrual Cycle: _____

14. Sexuality: _____

15. Emotional and Mental Health: _____

    _____

16. Substance Use: _____

17. Environment: _____

FOCUS ON DAYS 2, 21

21-Day Time Commitments

I commit myself to carrying out the activities of the 21-Day Program at the following times each day:

Meals: _____

Breakfast: _____

Lunch: _____

Dinner: _____

Exercise: _____

Evening Activity: _____

Journal Entry: _____

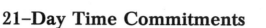

After you have completed this Goal Setting and Time Commitment process, I encourage you to reward yourself with a relaxing aromatherapy bath. Look through the bath recipes on pages 152 through 158 and choose one that appeals to you. As you relax in your bath, congratulate yourself! You have just made a major commitment to becoming the very best you can be. This goal-setting process is a first positive step toward cleansing and nourishing your body, mind, and emotions. Without thinking in detail about your specific goals, let the aromatic fumes of the essential oils subtly influence your mood. Absorb the wonderful combination of fragrances through all your senses. Fill yourself with thoughts of anticipation and optimism as you embark on the Clean and Clear Diet. The diet alone will immediately begin to give you an energetic, buoyant feeling, freeing your potential for creativity and loving self-expression. It will inspire you to do all of the healing activities in the 21-Day Cleansing and Rejuvenation Program.

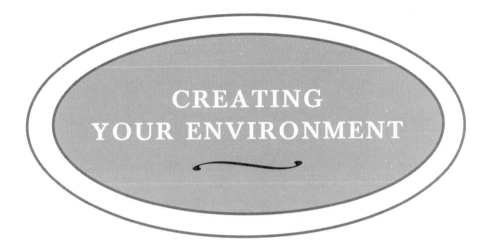

CREATING YOUR ENVIRONMENT

*T*his chapter is intended to support you in recreating your entire environment—body, mind and spirit—so that you are truly prepared to do the 21–Day Cleansing and Rejuvenation Program. By setting up your environment consciously, you will be more successful with your program.

YOUR PERSONAL SUPPORT SYSTEM

Sustenance from your friends or family is key when you commit yourself to a program of intensive whole–body cleansing. I encourage you to go on the program with a partner. You can create a buddy–support system, arranging for someone you can call on to share your experiences. You may want to surprise a close friend with a copy of this book, and then plan to do the program together. If you have a family, share your plans to do this program with your parents, your spouse, and your children. Hopefully, they will understand and support your commitment to improve your health and vitality—to be the very best you can be, for them and for yourself.

Human nature being what it is, some people will simply not support your efforts to improve yourself. They may discourage you or tease you, and make you feel self–conscious. Reduce the negativity in your life during this time. Share your plans only with positive, loving, upbeat people who will make you feel good about the new direction your life is taking.

Many of my clients like to keep a journal during the twenty–one days of mind/body cleansing. After your evening bath, when you get into bed, is a good time to take a moment and write down any thoughts or impressions that may have come to mind. What were the high points and the low points of the day? What new discoveries did you make? How are you feeling about your body? Have you found any new ways to deal with stress? You may make these observations in any form you choose—journal notes, drawings or poetic affirmations. By recording your personal experiences on a daily basis, you are supporting yourself and reinforcing your twenty–one–day commitment.

FITTING THE AT–HOME PROGRAM INTO YOUR LIFE

Many people spend a great deal of time and money on extended stays at health spas. Part of the reason they do this is because the spa environment eliminates the distractions of everyday life. One of the advantages of my 21–Day Program is that you can enjoy the personal benefits of a spa while you carry on with your normal life. You can continue to eat in restaurants, you can continue to socialize with friends, you can still take care of your family and loved ones, and you can continue to go to work.

During your goal setting on pages 25 through 30, I ask you to commit yourself to a schedule for the regular activities in this program—mealtimes, exercise, evening activities, bathing, and writing in your journal. Arrange plenty of private time for yourself on weekends for the extended sessions in your cleansing program. I know there will be special dates you just won't want to miss, or meetings you must attend. However, concentration and personal commitment are essential, so look at your schedule and pledge the necessary time to yourself!

Take a deep, self–indulgent breath—relax and enjoy yourself. My 21–Day Program is designed to be fun—three weeks of self–awareness and new approaches to things you do every day. I do not encourage extremism. Do not feel you must give up forever the things you enjoy. I encourage my clients to enjoy life, to be happy. I have developed a moderate cleansing program that everyone can feel comfortable with. I assure you that there is room in this program for variation, and I will help you to discover where you need to make adjustments in the recommended program to fit your personal energy level and emotional needs. One of my great personal lessons has been not to be hard on myself. If you go off the program, please take it with good humor. Just give a little shrug, forgive yourself, and get back on. Be gentle with yourself, and do the best you can. I promise you will still get great results!

CREATING YOUR AT–HOME SPA ENVIRONMENT

These activities are designed to set the scene and the mood for your 21–Day Program. Before you get into the actual 21–Day schedule, please look around your home—and particularly your bathroom—and think about what you can do to make it a more peaceful, nurturing, fun place to spend time in. You are embarking on a special program of taking care of yourself—a program just for you. Perhaps this is a good time to buy some fluffy new towels to enrich the experience of the wonderful baths, soaks, and steams that I will be showing you. You may want to buy colorful new sheets, or perhaps you would like to select some music, incense, or candles to create a meditative, peaceful atmosphere.

Now, go into your kitchen, open the cupboards, and remove all the things that will not be included in the 21–Day Program. Please remove the refined sugar, sugar syrups (except pure maple syrup), white flour, artificial creamers and sweeteners, candy, cookies, cakes, muffins, processed and canned foods, jams and jellies, raisins and other dried fruits, packaged cereals (except oatmeal), canned meats, bread, and crackers. If you plan to stop drinking coffee or alcohol during this program, get rid of them, too, although I am not insisting that you break your habits entirely.

I am not saying that you must never eat any of these foods again. If you decide to keep some of these items, simply pack them away in a box. If you are sharing your kitchen with your family or a friend, clear out a shelf in your cupboard and in your refrigerator for your own special foods.

Now, look in your refrigerator. Get rid of all the dairy products—cheese, milk, sour cream, and sweetened yogurts. You may keep a little butter if you wish, and you will be using plain yogurt for a facial this week. If you will not be tempted, you may keep the milk; I recommend using it in your bath on Day 8! Clean out the processed meats, red meats, sodas, and diet sodas. Remember, I am not saying that you must never eat cheese again, or never eat another lamb chop. The 21–Day Program will teach you how to incorporate such foods into your lifelong diet, but for the next three weeks I want you to start with a clean slate and reeducate yourself. Now, pack up all these things and donate them to a worthy cause, or store them away out of sight. Your kitchen is now clean and clear.

Please review the entire shopping list beginning on page 38 so you will know what kinds of foods, supplies, and equipment you will need. Some of the items on the shopping list may sound strange to you. Trust me; they will all be explained and enjoyed as we go through the program together.

You will probably need to visit more than one store to complete your shopping. Some supermarkets now have health–food sections, and you may be able to find many of the items there. If you have a health–food store in your area, it is more likely that you will find the organically grown fruits and vegetables that I recommend available there. Seeds, nuts, grains, and herbs will probably be available in bulk at the health–food store, too.

I am assuming that you already have a number of kitchen appliances, such as a blender or a coffee grinder. All such items needed for this program are listed under Equipment Inventory on the shopping list on page 39.

When you return from shopping be sure to store your food properly. Keep your oils in their glass bottles in a cool, dark place. Grains, seeds, and nuts should be stored in airtight glass (or less desirably, plastic) containers. Seaweed can be stored as it comes, in its package. Herbs should be stored in airtight containers, preferably glass ones. Tofu should be removed from the water it is packed in, and rinsed with fresh purified water every day. Store fruits and vegetables as you would normally do. On page 88 I will show you a Cleansing Soak for Fruits and Vegetables that will not only remove contaminants from any nonorganic produce, but will also increase its storage life.

PERSONALIZING YOUR SCHEDULE

The schedule provided for each day of the 21–Day Program must be personalized to your own requirements. You need to decide at what time you will eat your meals, do your exercise, perform your evening activities, and write in your journal. Of course, you may need to make some adjustments, but it is important that you make a commitment to set aside time each day to do all the scheduled activities.

Reading

Each day during the first week of the program and at least once a week for the second and third weeks, read the background information provided in Chapters 8 through 20. This will remind you of the benefits of doing the scheduled activities. Please, do not read the material at meals, since I want you to relax and eat slowly without distractions. A good idea is to pour yourself a cup of Inner Beauty Herbal Tea and sip it while you read the pertinent chapters. Consider reading before or after breakfast, during your afternoon break, or before bedtime.

Meals

It is important to space your meals at specific intervals, so that you can derive the greatest nutritional benefit from your food and allow your system to cleanse itself. The 21–Day Program is built around three meals a day, with midmorning and midafternoon snacks if you feel your energy flagging.

Exercise

Every day of your 21–Day Program you will do at least thirty minutes of brisk walking or other vigorous exercise. If you are exercising regularly at present, you already have an exercise schedule. If not, think about what time of day you would most enjoy taking a thirty-minute walk. You may decide to gradually increase your exercise time during the course of the program, but for now simply commit yourself to a half hour of exercise daily. Each day you will also be given a warm–up or stretch to precede your exercise schedule.

Evening Activities

Each evening, your 21–Day Program will provide special activities that are fun, relaxing, and rejuvenating. Your evening schedule may vary, but you will need to commit about an hour a night to your evening activity and your bath. Because these activities have a relaxing and stress–relieving effect, I recommend that you do them right before bedtime. I understand that there will be nights when this will not be possible, but it is very important for you to go through the learning experience that each of these evening activities provides. Think ahead now, and decide on an alternate time (such as right after work, or early in the morning) that you will be able to commit, when necessary, to each day's special practices.

Journal Entries

Sometimes you will be asked to write in your journal in the course of reading a chapter, or during an evening activity. Besides these self–affirmation exercises, I want you to make regular daily notes about the feelings that occur to you during the day. A convenient time to make such journal entries is right at bedtime, but some people may prefer to make their entries on rising in the morning, during a morning commute, or at some other time during the day when they are free of distractions. To help establish a regular habit of writing in your journal, commit yourself now to a time that you think will be best for you.

RELIEVING CLEANSING REACTIONS

As you begin to eat a lighter, fiber–rich diet and to cleanse your body of the toxins and waste that have accumulated over years of abuse, clogging up your systems of elimination, you may notice certain symptoms that can be annoying or even uncomfortable–headaches, skin eruptions or other blemishes, coated tongue, low energy, grouchiness or anger, and cold or flu–like symptoms such as a runny nose or body aches. These reactions occur because the toxins are being released from the cells and dumped into your system.

Do not be disturbed if some or all of these minor symptoms appear during the course of your cleansing program. Welcome them as a good sign; they are telling you that your body is really freeing itself of wastes and toxins that may have been stored in the cells and tissues for a long time. Any minor discomfort that you experience now means that you will have fewer problems in the future. Be sure to drink plenty of liquids and get adequate sleep to help your body deal with the added stress of removing these toxic substances.

I am stressing the intense use of cleansing preparations which flush the systems of elimination in order to help you get through these cleansing reactions as quickly and comfortably as possible. This is also why it is important for you to do colon cleansing during this program. If you do not remove the toxins promptly from the system, they will be reabsorbed.

In addition to the cleansing beverages in the schedule, be sure to drink plenty of the Hydrating Drink on page 81. Make it a habit to drink this sweetened water on arising, throughout the day, and before bedtime.

The granulated lecithin you will add to your protein drinks will help to minimize cleansing reactions by emulsifying toxins and flushing them out of your body. If you do have uncomfortable symptoms, take three 1200–milligram lecithin capsules with a cup of black tea (the small amount of caffeine in the tea serves as a carrier for the lecithin). Lecithin helps to detoxify the liver, so it will help to relieve symptoms without interfering with the cleansing process. Additional daily colon cleansing will also be helpful in keeping symptoms to a minimum. Some people may be bothered by bad breath or offensive body odor as part of their cleansing reaction. Remember that chlorophyll–rich vegetable juices can help. Refer to the list of Cleansing Juice Blends on page 110 for fresh green vegetables that help to eliminate unpleasant body odors.

As you progress though the 21 days of the program, you will be cleansing all your systems of elimination. Your daily skin brushing will remove dead cells and waste that are being eliminated through the skin. You will also use several special cleansing baths and steams that speed the elimination of toxins from your system. Every morning when you brush your teeth, also be sure to brush your tongue, to remove the buildup of waste that has coated it during the night. Tongue cleaning is an ancient custom in India. Be sure not to swallow the residue you remove from your tongue; rinse your mouth thoroughly with clean purified water.

If you should get blemishes or other skin eruptions as part of your cleansing reaction, please do not resort to chemical–laden cosmetics to mask the problem. It is perfectly all right to use cosmetics made of all–natural products to cover up any blemishes. Do promote the proper functioning of your skin by keeping it absolutely clean, and by getting plenty of exercise to promote sweating. The simple complexion–enhancing facials you will use during your evening activities will also help to cleanse and tone your skin without the use of synthetic products.

Massage will aid in flushing the toxins out of your system. You will perform both the Lower–Body Lymph Massage on page 162 and the Upper–Body Lymph Massage on page 163. You can also use the Quick Oriental Massage Remedies on page 175 for help with specific problems such as headache or low energy.

Rely on affirmations to reinforce your resolve as you deal with uncomfortable cleansing reactions–"I welcome this sign that my body is cleansing itself of waste and poisons," and "Each day my body is becoming cleaner and younger inside, as my cells are being rejuvenated."

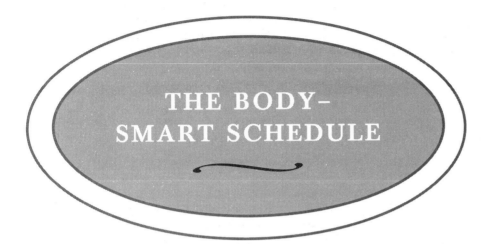

THE BODY–SMART SCHEDULE

Your First Week

The Cleansing and Rejuvenation Program has three phases. During the first, or elimination phase, you will begin to clean out your body by eliminating sources of toxins in your diet, concentrating on whole, organic foods and clean, pure water. As you eliminate sources of toxicity, you will gradually develop positive new habits as you begin to make the best possible use of exercise, breathing, bathing, and massage to promote cleansing, rejuvenation, beauty, and a feeling of vitality.

You will experience many techniques for promoting the correct functioning of your systems of elimination. You will begin to use special beverages to initiate a cleansing of your internal organs. You will begin to use exercise to stimulate blood and lymph flow and to encourage your skin to excrete waste through sweating. You will practice breathing exercises to help you cleanse your blood and lungs of waste, and use Inspirol (a cleansing inhalant) to clear your breathing passages. You will learn several stretching exercises based on yoga to stimulate the organs of elimination, and massage techniques to move the lymph, enhance blood circulation, and release tension. You will do dry–brush massage and prepare a variety of stimulating and cleansing baths to promote the eliminative function of the skin and lymph.

Try to begin your 21–Day Program when you have the free time necessary to properly prepare your environment, as I describe in Chapter 6. For

WEEK ONE

most people, beginning on a weekend will provide that opportunity. A well-organized beginning will assure you of greater success on the program.

Remember, you don't have to do it perfectly to get great results. Each time I do a Cleansing and Rejuvenation Program, I do it a bit differently; yet, I always achieve fantastic results. For example, if you have less time on any particular evening, simply do your aromatherapy bath! The additional evening activities will certainly enhance the results you achieve on that day and are very beneficial, but skipping them for one day will not diminish the overall results of the 21–Day Program.

Shopping List and Inventory: Week 1

This week's shopping list includes all breakfasts and special beverages, all ingredients needed to make Potassium Broth, and all ingredients for the beauty treatments. I have prepared this list assuming that you will be making all of your meals at home. However, for those of you who eat some of your meals out, be sure to check your daily schedules and refer to the indicated recipes, so that you can buy only the fresh ingredients you will need for lunches and dinners you actually do prepare at home. The Equipment Inventory lists equipment you will need this week.

NUTS, GRAINS, AND CEREALS

Almonds, 1/2 pound
Barley, 3 pounds
Millet, 2 pounds
Oatmeal, 1 pound

VEGETABLES OILS
(cold–pressed only)

Almond oil, 8 ounces
Olive oil, 16 ounces
Peanut oil, 8 ounces

FRUITS AND VEGETABLES
(organic, if possible)

Apples, 4
Beets, with tops, 2 bunches
Cantaloupe, 1
Carrots, with tops, 16
Celery, 2 bunches
Cucumber, 1
Garlic, 6 bulbs

Lemons, 4
Onions, 4
Orange, 1
Papaya, very ripe, 1
Parsley, 1 bunch
Pineapple, very ripe, 1
Potatoes, baking, 4
Raspberries, 1 pint basket, OR
   blueberries, 1 pint basket
Strawberries, 1 pint basket
Summer squash, 3
Zucchini, 4

BEVERAGES AND
MISCELLANEOUS FOODS

Apple juice, organic, 32 ounces, or
   pure maple syrup, 8 ounces
Milk, 1 quart
Water, bottled if you do not have a
   water purifier, 3 gallons
Yogurt, plain, low–fat, 1/2 pint

HERBS, SUPPLEMENTS, AND HEALTH–CARE ITEMS

You may puchase most of these items at your local health–food store or consult your Source Guide for ordering information.

Aloe vera juice, 1 quart
Body brush, vegetable bristle, 1
Body soap, nonchemical
Castor oil, 8 ounces
Dried Herbs:
    alfalfa, dried, 2 ounces
    cayenne pepper, 2 ounces
    mustard powder, 4 ounces
    oat straw, dried, 2 ounces
    peppermint leaves, dried, 4
      ounces
    sage, dried, 2 ounces
Epsom salts, two 4–pound boxes
Essential Oils:
    basil, chamomile, clary, sage,
    eucalyptus, lavender, marjo-
    ram, orange, peppermint,
    rose (or blended rose) rose
    geranium, rosemary, sandal-
    wood
Hydrogen peroxide, 3 percent
    solution, 1 small bottle
Loofa mitt, 1
NaPCA moisturizing spray
Sea–algae shower gel
Sea salt, 9 pounds
Sea sponge, soft, 1
Supplements:
    Coenzyme Q10, 30 mil-
    ligrams, 20 tablets
    Emergen–C, 36 packets, OR
      powdered vitamin C (ascor
      bic acid), 1 bottle

Vitamin E, 400 IU plus
    selenium, dry form, 60
    tablets
Germanium, capsules,
    powdered or sublingual
    form, 1 gram (due to FDA
    regulations this may not
    always be available)
Ginkgo–leaf extract, 40 mil
    ligrams, 20 tablets
Lecithin, granulated, 1
    pound, OR
Lecithin supplement,
    1,200 milligrams, 380
    capsules
Liquid chlorophyl, 1 8 ounce
    bottle
minerals, liquid, 1 quart
multivitamin supplement, 1
    month's supply
Omega–3 (EPA oil
    supplement), 1,000
    milligrams, 20 capsules
Omega–6 (GLA oil supple
    ment), 90 milligrams, 20
    capsules
Wheat–germ oil, 4 ounces
Witch hazel, 1 small bottle

EQUIPMENT INVENTORY

Blender
Coffee grinder or seed mill
Journal, blank
Mini–trampoline
Slant board
Tape recorder
Tub or bucket, small, for foot
    soaks
Vaporizer OR electric frying
    pan

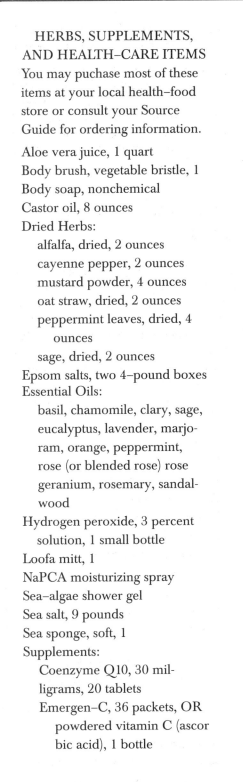

WEEK ONE

SATURDAY: DAY 1

MORNING ACTIVITY: Read Chapters 8 through 20 (pages 61 to 211).

AFTERNOON ACTIVITY: Clean out your kitchen (page 33). Review the Shopping List and Inventory: Week One (pages 38 to 39), Schedules for Days 1 through 7, and The Body-Smart Recipes (pages 79 to 110). Go shopping and store food.

EVENING ACTIVITY: Stress-Reduction Evening; Yoga Stress Releasers (page 124); follow with Stress Reduction Bath (page 155).

SUNDAY: DAY 2

MORNING CLEANSING: Warm shower. Scrub with a loofa mitt, using Seaweed Shower Gel. Follow with fifteen seconds of cool water.

MORNING ACTIVITY: Food and Beverage Preparation: Prepare and drink HOT LEMON-WATER FLUSH (page 80). Prepare INNER BEAUTY HERBAL TEA (page 81) and drink one cup at a time throughout the day between meals. Prepare HYDRATING DRINK (page 81) and drink it throughout the day between meals. Use CLEANSING SOAK FOR PRODUCE for any nonorganic fruits and vegetables (page 88). Prepare POTASSIUM BROTH (page 92).

AFTERNOON ACTIVITY: Self-Evaluation: Review your ORIENTATION QUESTIONNAIRE (page 14 to 19) and TOXICITY SYMPTOM CHECKLIST.

EXERCISE: Take a brisk walk for thirty minutes. Pay attention to your surroundings and your breathing.

DINNER: Nonprotein dinner: POTASSIUM BROTH (page 92), as much as you want. Combine with pasta or potatoes, and salad or vegetables.

EVENING ACTIVITY: Goal Setting: Review your 21-DAY GOALS CONTRACT (page 29). Complete 21-DAY TIME COMMITMENTS (page 30). Follow with INSPIRATION BATH (page 155).

MONDAY: DAY 3

ON AWAKENING: One 8-ounce glass of HOT LEMON-WATER FLUSH (page 80). Prepare your INNER BEAUTY HERBAL TEA (page 81); drink one cup at a time between meals throughout the day.

MORNING CLEANSING: Using a loofa mitt, scrub the entire body using a nonsoap cleanser, such as Sea-algae Shower Gel, while showering with hot water. End with thirty seconds of cold water.

BREAKFAST: FRESH APPLE BREAKFAST (page 89).

MIDMORNING SNACK: Optional Protein Drink–SESAME–SEED MILK (page 108).

LUNCH: Fish, chicken, or tofu with steamed or raw vegetables.

DINNER: YAM DELIGHT (page 95); SUPER SALAD (page 98) with FAT–LOSS DRESSING of your choice (pages 100 to 101).

EXERCISE: Precede exercise with OXYGENATION COCKTAIL (page 82). Then take a walk for thirty minutes. Maintain a brisk, steady pace, paying attention to your surroundings and your breathing.

EVENING ACTIVITY: CUCUMBER CLEANSING FACIAL (page 146). Remove facial and apply the YOGURT TONING MASK (page 147), which is kept on during the TRANQUILITY BATH (page 156).

TUESDAY: DAY 4

ON AWAKENING: One 8–ounce glass of HOT LEMON–WATER FLUSH (page 80). Prepare INNER BEAUTY HERBAL TEA (page 81); drink throughout the day between meals.

MORNING CLEANSING: Alternating Hot and Cold Shower–begin with three to five minutes of hot water; switch to ten to fifteen seconds of cold water. Repeat three times, ending with cold water. Dry briskly with a coarse towel.

BREAKFAST: SLICED FRESH PINEAPPLE (page 90).

MIDMORNING SNACK: Optional Protein Drink–ALMOND MILK (page 108).

LUNCH: Fish, chicken, or tofu with steamed or raw vegetables.

DINNER: SQUASH BISQUE (page 94); SUPER SALAD (page 98) with FAT–LOSS DRESSING of your choice (pages 100 to 101).

EXERCISE: Precede exercise with OXYGENATION COCKTAIL (page 82). WAKE–UP SHAKE–UP (page 116), followed by brisk walking for thirty minutes using MEDITATIVE WALKING BREATH (page 120).

EVENING ACTIVITY: ANTIGRAVITY TONE–UP (page 122), followed by DEEP HEAT BATH (page 157).

WEDNESDAY:DAY 5

ON AWAKENING: One 8–ounce glass of HOT LEMON–WATER FLUSH (page 80). Prepare INNER BEAUTY HERBAL TEA (page 81); drink throughout the day between meals. Prepare REJUVELAC (page 88).

MORNING CLEANSING: DRY BRUSH MASSAGE (page 144). Follow with a hot shower, finishing with a thirty–second cold splash.

BREAKFAST: PAPAYA COMPLEXION BREAKFAST (page 90).

MIDMORNING SNACK: Optional Protein Drink–SUNFLOWER–SEED MILK (page 109).

LUNCH: Fish, chicken, or tofu with steamed or raw vegetables.

DINNER: CAULIFLOWER BISQUE (page 95). SUPER SALAD (page 98) with FAT–LOSS DRESSING of your choice (pages 100 to 101).

EXERCISE: Precede exercise with OXYGENATION COCKTAIL (page 82). DANCER'S WARM–UP (page 117) followed by REBOUNDING WORKOUT (page 120) for ten to twenty minutes, or walking for twenty to thirty minutes.

EVENING ACTIVITY: HOT FOOT SOAK (page 162), followed by LOWER–BODY LYMPHATIC MASSAGE (page 162). Drink one cup REJUVELAC (page 88).

THURSDAY: DAY 6

ON AWAKENING: One 8–ounce glass of HOT LEMON–WATER FLUSH (page 80). Prepare INNER BEAUTY HERBAL TEA (page 81); drink throughout the day between meals. Use INSPIROL (Cleansing Inhalant) (page 135).

MORNING CLEANSING: Hot shower followed by FRICTION AIR BATH (page 146).

BREAKFAST: BERRY BREAKFAST (page 91).

MIDMORNING SNACK: Optional Protein Drink–SESAME-SEED MILK (page 108).

LUNCH: Fish, chicken, or tofu with steamed or raw vegetables.

DINNER: HIGH–IRON SALAD (page 99); steamed mixed vegetables with TOFU–MISO TOPPING (page 105).

EXERCISE: Precede exercise with OXYGENATION COCKTAIL (page

82). DANCER'S WARM–UP (page 117), followed by YOGIC SWIM-MING (page 125) for twelve to twenty minutes; or brisk walking for thirty minutes.

EVENING ACTIVITY: Use INSPIROL (Cleansing Inhalant) (page 135); follow with THREE–PART BREATHING (page 137), COMPLETE BREATH (page 138), and ALTERNATE–HEMISPHERE BREATHING (page 139). Take the SEA–MINERAL BATH (page 154). Drink one cup Rejuvelac (page 139).

FRIDAY: DAY 7

ON AWAKENING: One 8–ounce glass of HOT LEMON–WATER FLUSH (page 80). Prepare INNER BEAUTY HERBAL TEA (page 81); drink throughout the day between meals. Use INSPIROL (Cleansing Inhalant) (page 135). Pour off today's REJUVELAC (page 88). Drink one cup and save the rest. Prepare another batch for tomorrow.

MORNING CLEANSING: MORNING COLD SPLASH AND RUB (page 154).

BREAKFAST: FRESH CANTALOUPE BREAKFAST (page 91).

MIDMORNING SNACK: Optional Protein Drink–ALMOND MILK (page 108).

LUNCH: Fish, chicken, or tofu with steamed or raw vegetables.

DINNER: Baked potato with GREEN GODDESS TOPPING (page 102); sauteed mixed vegetables.

EXERCISE: Precede exercise with OXYGENATION COCKTAIL (page 82). Warm up with YOGA SELF–MASSAGE (page 126), follow with thirty minutes of brisk walking.

EVENING ACTIVITY: Drink one cup of REJUVELAC. Add the remainder to tonight's bath. ANTIGRAVITY FACIAL MASSAGE (page 174), followed by WARM SOAK AND STROKE (page 177).

WEEK ONE

WEEK TWO

Tonight marks the end of the first week of your 21–Day Cleansing and Rejuvenation Program. Your body is building new cells, and your systems of elimination are working more efficiently to keep your tissues and body fluids clean and clear. Many of the toxins and wastes stored in your body have been released and eliminated. As you lie in bed relaxing after your Warm Soak and Stroke, take time to be aware of your body. Breathe deeply and notice any changes that have occurred since you began the program.

Do you feel more energetic, less achy, lighter, and more limber? Draw your breath into every part of your body, noticing any areas that seem sore or tense. As you exhale, breathe out the tension and notice the wonderful feeling of cleanliness and relaxation produced by your bath and massage. Let go of all your stress, negativity, and doubts tonight. Tomorrow you will be moving on to new challenges as you enter a new, more intense phase of your cleansing program

*Y*OUR *S*ECOND *W*EEK

This week you will begin the intensified cleansing phase of the 21–Day Program. Every meal, every beverage, every activity, is designed to gently flush and cleanse your organs, tissues, and cells. Even your thoughts and feelings will take on a renewed brightness and clarity.

Last week you prepared yourself for cleansing by following the Clean and Clear Diet, which eliminated unnecessary contaminants and congesting foods, and taught you how to combine foods properly so that they would not leave behind undigested wastes in your system. This week's diet eliminates animal protein and focuses on simple, cleansing foods. Your daily menus will progress from a combination of cooked and raw fruits and vegetables to raw foods only. The final two days you will be on a fast of juices and thin vegetable broth. This progressively lighter diet leading to a liquid fast is designed to give your systems of elimination a deep rest and allow them to release the toxins and wastes they have accumulated. This cleansing process will be assisted by a variety of new beverages to flush your body. You will also prepare special detoxifying baths and experience techniques for colon cleansing.

During this deep cleansing phase you will be clearing your body of wastes much more intensely. You will be eliminating many of the foods to which people are often unknowingly sensitive. You may experience some minor symptoms, such as a light headache or a pimple or two, as your body begins to throw off the toxins that are being released from the cells. Your body will become progressively cleaner, clearer, and lighter. You will discover that the cleansing process is not only physical but also psychological. Often, as people clean out their bodies, they find that they are also releasing long–held emotions that have been held in the abdominal area, and they may experience profound personal insights. In working with my clients, I have been amazed to see how the cleansing process brings the mind and body into greater harmony.

Although this week's program may appear rigorous at first glance, your daily diet and activities will be similar to those you would be following at an exclusive spa. Yet you will still be able to go to work, socialize with friends, eat meals out, take care of your family and your personal needs–with the increased energy and an enhanced sense of well–being. And best of all, you will discover revitalizing life–extension techniques to integrate into your daily life.

This week's therapeutic cleansing regimen is not the sort of program you would follow all the time, but it does contain rejuvenation and weight–loss techniques that you will be able to use both for periodic touch–ups and for special health boosts in the future.

Shopping List and Inventory: Week 2

This week's shopping list includes all breakfasts, special beverages, and the basic ingredients for protein drinks. Please check your daily schedules and refer to the indicated recipes so that you can buy the fresh ingredients and staples you will need for the meals you will prepare at home. If you need to make fresh juices with a juicer, check the recipes for Cleansing Juice Blends to determine what additional vegetables you will need. If you are making more Potassium Broth, replenish your supply of ingredients. Check the items marked with an asterisk and replenish them if necessary up to the quantity indicated. The Equipment Inventory lists equipment you will need for this week's activities.

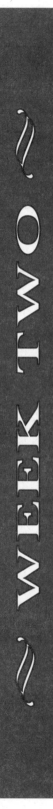

WEEK TWO

NUTS, GRAINS, AND CEREALS

Almonds, 1 pound
Barley, 2 pounds
Sesame seeds, 1/2 pound
Sunflower seeds, shelled,
    unsalted, 1-1/2 pounds

FRUITS AND VEGETABLES
(organic, if possible)

Cucumber, 1
Garlic, 3 bulbs
Ginger, fresh, 1 large piece
Lemons, 6
Oranges, 3
Papaya, very ripe, 1
Pineapple, very ripe, 1

VEGETABLES OILS
(cold-pressed only)

Safflower oil, 16 ounces

BEVERAGES AND MISCELLANEOUS FOODS

Apple juice, organic, 32 ounces
Carob powder, 2 ounces
Eggs (for facials), 6
Milk (for eye packs), 1 pint
Tahini, 1-pound can
Water, bottled if you do not
    have a water purifier,
    3 gallons

HERBS, SUPPLEMENTS, AND HEALTH-CARE ITEMS

You may puchase most of these items at your local health-food store or consult your Source Guide for ordering information.

Baking soda, 16 ounces
Castor oil, 1 small bottle
Cotton balls, sterile, small box
Dried Herbs:
    chaparral, dried, 2 ounces
    fennel seeds, 1 ounces
    fenugreek seeds, 1 ounce
    flax seeds, powdered,
        3 ounces
    juniper berries, 1 ounce
    licorice root, 2 ounces
    parsley root, 1 ounce
    peppermint leaves, dried,
        2 ounces
    psyllium seeds, powdered,
        3 ounces
    uva-ursi leaves, 1 ounce
Epsom salts, 4 pounds
Essential Oil: juniper
Petroleum jelly or lubricating
  (K-Y brand) jelly

EQUIPMENT INVENTORY

Balloons, thick, 1 dozen
Electric heating pad
Enema bag
Flannel, soft wool, piece (16
    inches wide by 12 to 18
    inches long)
Garbage bag or dry cleaner's
    bag, plastic, large
Juicer (optional)

SATURDAY:DAY 8

ON AWAKENING: One 8–ounce glass of HOT LEMON–WATER FLUSH (page 80). Prepare INNER BEAUTY HERBAL TEA WITH CHAPARRAL (page 84); drink throughout the day between meals. Use INSPIROL (Cleansing Inhalant) (page 135).

MORNING CLEANSING: DRY BRUSH MASSAGE (page 144). Follow with Alternating Hot and Cold Shower–begin with three to five minutes of hot water; switch to ten to fifteen seconds of cold water. Repeat three times, ending with cold water. Dry briskly with a coarse towel.

BREAKFAST: SLICED FRESH PINEAPPLE BREAKFAST (page 90).

MIDMORNING SNACK: CARROT SHAKE (page 110) based on seed or nut milk of choice. Add one tablespoon of granulated lecithin.

LUNCH: Steamed mixed vegetables with GOLDEN GODDESS TOPPING (page 102).

MIDAFTERNOON SNACK: Optional–CARROT SHAKE (page 110) or REJUVELAC (page 88), one cup.

AFTERNOON ACTIVITIES: Shop for week's food and supplies, see SHOPPING LIST AND INVENTORY: WEEK 2 (page 46) and SCHEDULES for Days 8 through 14. Use CLEANSING SOAK FOR FRUITS AND VEGETABLES (page 88) for nonorganic produce. Prepare barley water for CLEOPATRA'S MILK BATH (page 158); make four times the recipe. Use one cup tonight, and freeze the other three in separate containers for later in the program. Prepare POTASSIUM BROTH (page 92) for the week; refrigerate two batches of thick bisque for tonight and Sunday and freeze two batches of thin broth for later this week. (If you have any Potassium Broth left from Week 1, adjust the size of this week's recipe accordingly.)

DINNER: CARROT BISQUE (page 95), as much as you wish. Make the bisque with thick potassium broth. Add one tablespoon of granulated lecithin.

EXERCISE: Precede exercise with OXYGENATION COCKTAIL (page 82), follow with LYMPH–CLEANSING WARM–UP (page 118) and thirty minutes of brisk walking or twenty minutes of REBOUNDING WORKOUT (page 120).

EVENING ACTIVITY: Drink one cup of REJUVELAC (page 88). Add the remainder to tonight's bath. TUMMY MASSAGE (page 187). Follow with CLEOPATRA'S MILK BATH (page 158); while in bath apply MILK EYE PACKS (page 147). Just before going to bed, do ALTERNATE–HEMISPHERE BREATHING (page 139) and take INTESTINAL CLEANSER (page 87).

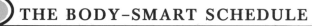

SUNDAY:DAY 9

ON AWAKENING: One 8-ounce glass of HOT LEMON-WATER FLUSH (page 80). Prepare INNER BEAUTY HERBAL TEA WITH CHAPARRAL (page 84); drink throughout the day between meals. Use INSPIROL (Cleansing Inhalant) (page 135).

MORNING CLEANSING: DRY BRUSH MASSAGE (page 144), followed by warm shower.

BREAKFAST: PAPAYA COMPLEXION BREAKFAST (page 90).

MIDMORNING SNACK: HOT MOCK CHOCOLATE (page 109) based on seed or nut milk of choice. Add one tablespoon of granulated lecithin.

LUNCH: Steamed mixed vegetables with TAHINI-TOFU TOPPING (page 104).

MIDAFTERNOON SNACK: Optional–HOT MOCK CHOCOLATE (page 109) or REJUVELAC (page 88), one cup.

DINNER: CAULIFLOWER BISQUE (page 95), as much as you wish. Make the bisque with thick potassium broth. Add one tablespoon of granulated lecithin to the bisque.

EXERCISE: Precede exercise with OXYGENATION COCKTAIL (page 82), BALLOON BREATHING (page 135) and LYMPH-CLEANSING WARM-UP (page 118) and thirty minutes of brisk walking or twenty minutes of REBOUNDING WORKOUT (page 146).

EVENING ACTIVITY: Drink one cup of REJUVELAC (page 88). Apply EGG-YOLK MASK (page 146) to face, leave on while doing DIGESTION TONING POSTURES (page 128). Follow with AROMATIC FUME BATH with Witch Hazel (page 152). Take INTESTINAL CLEANSER (page 87).

MONDAY: DAY 10

ON AWAKENING: One 8-ounce glass of HYDRATING DRINK (page 81). Prepare HERBAL PURIFICATION TEA for the day (page 84). Use INSPIROL (Cleansing Inhalant) (page 135). Prepare protein drink for midday snacks.

MORNING CLEANSING: DRY BRUSH MASSAGE (page 144), followed by MORNING COLD SPLASH AND RUB (page 154).

BREAKFAST: LIVER FLUSH #1 (page 85). Follow with one cup of HERBAL PURIFICATION TEA; drink a second cup of the tea during the morning.

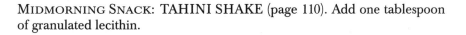

MIDMORNING SNACK: TAHINI SHAKE (page 110). Add one tablespoon of granulated lecithin.

LUNCH: SUPER SALAD (page 98) with FAT–LOSS DRESSING (pages 100 to 101) of choice. Sprinkle granulated lecithin on salad. If eating in a restaurant, order a raw–vegetable salad. Bring your own dressing or use olive oil and lemon juice.

MIDAFTERNOON SNACK: Optional–TAHINI SHAKE (page 110), or REJUVELAC (page 88), one cup. One hour before dinner, prepare and drink one cup of DIURETIC TEA (page 86).

DINNER: RAW–VEGETABLE DELIGHT (page 97), as much as you wish.

EXERCISE: Precede exercise with OXYGENATION COCKTAIL (page 82). LYMPH–CLEANSING WARM –UP (page 118) followed by thirty minutes of brisk walking or twenty minutes of REBOUNDING WORK-OUT (page 120).

EVENING ACTIVITY: Drink one cup of REJUVELAC (page 88). Add remainder to tonight's bath. UPPER–BODY LYMPH MASSAGE (page 163), follow with EPSOM SALTS SOAK with HYDRATING BATH SALTS (page 153). Accompany bath with EASY STEAM (page 152), using three drops of juniper essential oil. Drink one cup of HERBAL PURIFICA-TION TEA before going to bed. Take INTESTINAL CLEANSER (page 87).

TUESDAY: DAY 11

ON AWAKENING: One 8–ounce glass of HYDRATING DRINK (page 81). Prepare HERBAL PURIFICATION TEA for the day (page 84). Use INSPIROL (Cleansing Inhalant) (page 135). Prepare protein drink for mid-day snacks.

MORNING CLEANSING: Hot shower, finishing with a one–minute cold splash. Follow with DRY BRUSH MASSAGE (page 144).

BREAKFAST: LIVER FLUSH #2 (page 86). Follow with one cup of HERBAL PURIFICATION TEA. Drink a second cup of the tea during the morning.

MIDMORNING SNACK: CARROT SHAKE (page 110). Add one table-spoon of granulated lecithin.

LUNCH: SUPER SALAD (page 98) with FAT–LOSS DRESSING (pages 100 to 101) of choice. Sprinkle granulated lecithin on salad. If eating in a restaurant, order a raw–vegetable salad. Bring your own dressing or use olive oil and lemon juice.

WEEK TWO

MIDAFTERNOON SNACK: Optional–CARROT SHAKE (page 110), or REJUVELAC (page 88), one cup. One hour before dinner, prepare and drink one cup of DIURETIC TEA (page 86).

DINNER: RAW–VEGETABLE "CREAM" SOUP (page 97), as much as you wish.

EXERCISE: OXYGENATION COCKTAIL (page 82). LYMPH CLEAN-SING WARM–UP (page 118) followed by thirty minutes of brisk walking or twenty minutes of REBOUNDING WORKOUT (page 120).

EVENING ACTIVITY: Begin preparations for CHAPARRAL DETOXIFY-ING BATH (page 157). Drink one cup of REJUVELAC (page 88). Add remainder to tonight's bath. LOWER-BODY LYMPH MASSAGE (page 162), follow with CHAPARRAL DETOXIFYING BATH. Accompany bath with EASY STEAM (page 152), using three drops of your favorite essential oil. Drink one cup of HERBAL PURIFICATION TEA before going to bed. Take INTESTINAL CLEANSER (page 87).

WEDNESDAY: DAY 12

ON AWAKENING: Drink one 8–ounce glass of HYDRATING DRINK (page 81). Prepare HERBAL PURIFICATION TEA for the day (page 84). Use INSPIROL (Cleansing Inhalant) (page 135). Prepare protein drink for midday snacks.

MORNING CLEANSING: Warm shower followed by DRY BRUSH MAS-SAGE (page 144).

BREAKFAST: LIVER FLUSH #1 (page 85). Follow with one cup of HERBAL PURIFICATION TEA. Drink a second cup of the tea during the morning.

MIDMORNING SNACK: MAPLE NUT–SHAKE (page 109). Add one table-spoon of granulated lecithin.

LUNCH: SUPER SALAD (page 98) with SPA SALSA (page 103). Sprinkle granulated lecithin on salad. If eating in a restaurant, order a raw–vegetable salad. Bring your own dressing or use olive oil and lemon juice.

MIDAFTERNOON SNACK: Optional–MAPLE–NUT SHAKE (page 109), or REJUVELAC (page 88), one cup. One hour before dinner, prepare and drink one cup of DIURETIC TEA (page 86).

DINNER: RAW–VEGETABLE "CREAM" SOUP (page 97) with variation of choice, as much as you wish.

EXERCISE: OXYGENATION COCKTAIL (page 82). LYMPH CLEAN-SING WARM–UP (page 118), followed by thirty minutes of brisk walking or twenty minutes of REBOUNDING WORKOUT (page 120).

EVENING ACTIVITY: Drink one cup of REJUVELAC (page 88). Add the remainder to tonight's bath. Professional COLONIC IRRIGATION or a CLEANSING ENEMA (page 183) accompanied by TUMMY MASSAGE (page 187). Follow with CLEOPATRA'S MILK BATH (page 158). While in bath apply MILK EYE PACKS (page 147). Drink one cup of HERBAL PURIFICATION TEA before going to bed. Take INTESTINAL CLEANSER (page 87).

THURSDAY: DAY 13

ON AWAKENING: One 8–ounce glass of HYDRATING DRINK. Prepare HERBAL PURIFICATION TEA (page 84). Use INSPIROL (Cleansing Inhalant) (page 135). Prepare protein drink for midday snacks.

MORNING CLEANSING: DRY BRUSH MASSAGE (page 144). Follow with Alternating Hot and Cold Shower–begin with three to five minutes of hot water; switch to ten to fifteen seconds of cold water. Repeat three times, ending with cold water. Dry briskly with a coarse towel.

BREAKFAST: LIVER FLUSH #2 (page 86). Follow with one cup of HERBAL PURIFICATION TEA. Drink a second cup of the tea during the morning.

MIDMORNING SNACK: SESAME SEED SHAKE (page 108). Add one tablespoon of granulated lecithin.

LUNCH: CLEANSING JUICE BLEND (page 110), as much as you want.

MIDAFTERNOON SNACK: Optional–Eight ounces of CLEANSING JUICE BLEND (page 110) or REJUVELAC (page 88), one cup. One hour before dinner, prepare and drink one cup of DIURETIC TEA (page 86).

DINNER: POTASSIUM BROTH (page 92), as much as you wish. If desired for an extra boost, add Miso to taste, up to one teaspoon per cup.

EXERCISE: OXYGENATION COCKTAIL (page 82). LYMPH CLEANSING WARM-UP (page 118), followed by thirty minutes of brisk walking or twenty minutes of REBOUNDING WORKOUT (page 120).

EVENING ACTIVITY: Drink one cup of REJUVELAC (page 88). Add remainder to tonight's bath. Apply OATMEAL–EGG WHITE FACIAL (page 146); leave on while doing YOGA SELF–MASSAGE (page 126). Remove facial and take hot EPSOM SALTS SOAK (page 153). Accompany bath with EASY STEAM (page 152), using three drops of a favorite essential oil. Drink one cup of HERBAL PURIFICATION TEA before going to bed. Take INTESTINAL CLEANSER (page 87).

WEEK TWO

FRIDAY: DAY 14

ON AWAKENING: One 8-ounce glass of HYDRATING DRINK (page 81). Prepare HERBAL PURIFICATION TEA for the day (page 84). Use INSPIROL (Cleansing Inhalant) (page 135). Prepare protein drink for mid-day snacks.

MORNING CLEANSING: MORNING COLD SPLASH AND RUB (page 154), followed by DRY BRUSH MASSAGE (page 144).

BREAKFAST: LIVER FLUSH #1 (page 89). Follow with one cup of HERBAL PURIFICATION TEA. Drink a second cup of the tea during the morning.

MIDMORNING SNACK: CARROT SHAKE (page 110). Add one tablespoon of granulated lecithin.

LUNCH: CLEANSING JUICE BLEND of choice (page 110), as much as you want.

MIDAFTERNOON SNACK: Optional–Eight ounces of CLEANSING JUICE BLEND (page 110) or REJUVELAC (page 88), one cup. One hour before dinner, prepare and drink one cup of DIURETIC TEA (page 86).

DINNER: POTASSIUM BROTH (page 92), as much as you wish. If desired for an extra boost, add Miso to taste, up to one teaspoon per cup.

EXERCISE: OXYGENATION COCKTAIL (page 82). LYMPH CLEAN-SING WARM-UP (page 118), followed by thirty minutes of brisk walking or twenty minutes of REBOUNDING WORKOUT (page 120).

EVENING ACTIVITY: (At home night): Begin preparations for CHAPAR-RAL DETOXIFYING BATH (page 157). Drink one cup of REJUVELAC (page 88). Add remainder to tonight's bath. HOT CASTOR OIL ABDOM-INAL WRAP (page 186). While wrap is on, do THREE-PART BREATHING (page 137) and COMPLETE BREATH (page 138), and simply relax. Follow with CHAPARRAL DETOXIFYING BATH. Accompany bath with EASY STEAM (page 152), using three drops of another favorite essential oil. Drink one cup of HERBAL PURIFICATION TEA before going to bed. Take INTESTINAL CLEANSER (page 87).

WEEK TWO

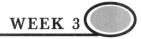

Congragulations! You have completed the most rigorous week of the Program. The goal of the 21–Day Program is to rid your body of toxins, awakening the sleeping beauty within you. This beauty may have been concealed by layers of internal pollution from years of incorrect eating, stress, and accumulated waste. Just as you have released the waste from your cells, tissues, and organs, you have also released negative emotional and mental patterns. The cleansing process brings body, mind, emotions, and spirit into greater harmony. Take time in your bath tonight to reflect on the lighter, clearer, and wonderfully rejuvenated feelings you are beginning to experience.

*Y*OUR *T*HIRD *W*EEK

You have arrived at the third and final week of your At–Home Program. If you have followed the program faithfully, I am sure you are now feeling wonderfully light and clear. I remember that when I first experimented with juice fasting many years ago, I was amazed at how dramatically different I felt. I experienced a sustained clarity of mind that was entirely new for me, and a constant flow of energy replaced my usual daily ups and downs. During the first two weeks of the 21–Day Program, you have eliminated the foods that generally cause people problems. This week, as you complete the intensive releasing and cleansing process of Week 2 and begin to add foods back, you have an opportunity to discover how these various foods may have been affecting you. I suggest that you pay careful attention to any cravings you may experience and watch how you feel as you reintroduce various foods back into your diet. By noticing how your body reacts, you will be able to find the foods that bring out the very best in you.

This week's diet plan returns gradually to the Clean and Clear Diet that you followed during Week 1. You will break your two day liquid fast with two days of raw fruits and vegetables, followed by two days of raw and cooked fruits and vegetables. As you return to regular eating, you will be practicing the proper techniques to keep your eliminative systems clean and clear, so that toxic waste never builds up in your system again. Unfortunately, we are not taught simple tools for cleansing in our culture.

Many of this week's activities are designed to teach you how to deal with constipation and cellulite once and for all! Did you know that laxatives are the best selling over–the–counter remedy in this country? Many people reading this book have suffered from constipation or poor elimination habits and may be seeking help for this problem. Constipation results in the buildup of toxic–waste material in your colon–wastes that are periodically absorbed into your body, aging it. During the Cleansing and Rejuvenation program you are learning how to get rid of this toxic waste and how to prevent it from building up in the future. This toxic waste is also a major factor in the formation of cellulite–those unattractive, lumpy deposits of fat, water, and waste that ruin many otherwise good figures. By learning how to avoid constipation forever, you will also learn how to keep cellulite from forming in your body. In addition, my cleansing program, along with special cellulite–reducing activities, will help you to reduce any cellulite you may now have.

Please remember, if you are experiencing uncomfortable cleansing reactions as I describe on page 35, I want you to do more than the recommended number of colon cleansings. At least one colon cleansing per day is recommended in many spas; it is the key to completely cleansing out your body.

Shopping List and Inventory: Week 3

This week's shopping list includes staple foods that you will need for the final week of the program, including all breakfasts, special beverages, and protein drinks. Please check your daily schedules and refer to the indicated recipes so that you can buy the fresh ingredients for the lunches and dinners you will prepare at home. If you are making more Potassium Broth, replenish your supply of ingredients. Check your stock of all items marked with an asterisk and replenish them if necessary up to the indicated quantity.

NUTS, GRAINS, AND CEREALS

Almonds, 1/2 pound
Barley, 1 pound
Sesame seeds, 1/2 pound
Sunflower seeds, shelled,
    unsalted, 1/2 pound

FRUITS AND VEGETABLES
(organic, if possible)

Apples, 4
Garlic, 3 bulbs
Grapes, 2 pounds
Lemons, 4
Papaya, very ripe, 1
Pineapple, very ripe, 1
Watermelon, 1/2

BEVERAGES AND MISCELLANEOUS FOODS

Apple juice, organic, 32 ounces
Apple–cider vinegar, 1 bottle
Milk (for eye packs), 1 pint
Water, bottled (if you do not have
    a water purifier), 3 gallons

HERBS, SUPPLEMENTS, AND HEALTH–CARE ITEMS

You may puchase these items at your local health–food store or consult your Source Guide for ordering information.

Honey, with royal jelly, 1 small jar
Essential Oil: geranium

SATURDAY: DAY 15

ON AWAKENING: One 8–ounce glass of HOT LEMON–WATER FLUSH (page 80); add one teaspoon honey with ROYAL JELLY (page 206). Prepare INNER BEAUTY HERBAL TEA (page 81); drink throughout the day between meals. Use INSPIROL (Cleansing Inhalant) (page 135). Prepare protein drink for midday snacks.

MORNING CLEANSING: Hot shower followed by FRICTION AIR BATH (page 146).

BREAKFAST: CLEANSING WATERMELON BREAKFAST (page 92).

MIDMORNING SNACK: TAHINI SHAKE (page 110). Add one tablespoon of granulated lecithin.

LUNCH: APPLE–CIDER VINEGAR DRINK (page 87), followed by SUPER SALAD (page 98) with SPA SALSA (page 103).

AFTERNOON ACTIVITIES: Shop for week's food and supplies, see SHOPPING LIST AND INVENTORY (page 54) and SCHEDULES for Days 15 through 21. Use CLEANSING SOAK FOR FRUITS AND VEGETABLES (page 88) for nonorganic produce. Prepare POTASSIUM BROTH (page 92) for the week. Refrigerate one batch of thick bisque for Monday, and freeze two 4–cup batches of thin broth for later this week. (If you have any Potassium Broth left from last week, adjust the size of this week's recipe accordingly.) Professional COLONIC IRRIGATION or CLEANSING ENEMA (page 188).

MIDAFTERNOON SNACK: Optional–TAHINI SHAKE (page 110) or REJUVELAC (page 88), one cup.

DINNER: RAW VEGETABLE DELIGHT (page 97), as much as you want.

EXERCISE: OXYGENATION COCKTAIL (page 82). WAKE–UP SHAKE–UP (page 116), followed by thirty minutes of brisk walking.

EVENING ACTIVITY: Drink one cup of REJUVELAC (page 88). Add the remainder to tonight's bath. THREE–PART BREATHING (page 137), COMPLETE BREATH (page 138), and ALTERNATE HEMISPHERE BREATHING (page 139). SEA SALT SCRUB (page 145), followed by a warm bath with EASY STEAM (page 152), using three drops of sandalwood (or your favorite) essential oil.

SUNDAY: DAY 16

ON AWAKENING: One 8–ounce glass of HOT LEMON–WATER FLUSH (page 80); add one teaspoon honey with ROYAL JELLY (page 206). Prepare INNER BEAUTY HERBAL TEA (page 81); drink throughout the day between meals. Use INSPIROL (Cleansing Inhalant) (page 135).

MORNING CLEANSING: DRY BRUSH MASSAGE (page 144). Follow with Alternating Hot and Cold Shower—begin with three to five minutes of hot water; switch to ten to fifteen seconds of cold water. Repeat three times, ending with cold water. Dry briskly with a coarse towel.

BREAKFAST: HEALING GRAPE BREAKFAST (page 89).

MIDMORNING SNACK: HOT MOCK CHOCOLATE (page 109). Add one tablespoon of granulated lecithin.

LUNCH: APPLE–CIDER VINEGAR DRINK (page 87), followed by SUPER SALAD (page 98) with FAT LOSS DRESSING (pages 100 to 101) of choice.

MIDAFTERNOON SNACK: Optional—HOT MOCK CHOCOLATE (page 109) or REJUVELAC (page 88), one cup.

AFTERNOON ACTIVITY: FATHER KNEIPP'S FOOTBATH (page 162) for twenty minutes, followed by Professional Massage, preferably in your home.

DINNER: Raw vegetable platter with GREEN GODDESS TOPPING (page 102).

EXERCISE: OXYGENATION COCKTAIL (page 82), DANCER'S WARM–UP (page 117) followed by thirty minutes of brisk walking.

EVENING ACTIVITY: Drink one cup of REJUVELAC (page 88). AROMATIC FUME BATH with Witch Hazel (page 152). YOGA ARCH POSE VARIATIONS (page 124), followed by YOGA STRESS RELEASERS (page 124), just before bedtime.

MONDAY: DAY 17

ON AWAKENING: One 8–ounce glass of HOT LEMON–WATER FLUSH (page 80); add one teaspoon honey with ROYAL JELLY (page 206). Prepare INNER BEAUTY HERBAL TEA (page 81); drink throughout the day between meals. Use INSPIROL (Cleansing Inhalant) (page 135).

MORNING CLEANSING: DRY BRUSH MASSAGE (page 144), followed by MORNING COLD SPLASH AND RUB (page 154).

BREAKFAST: PAPAYA COMPLEXION BREAKFAST (page 90).

MIDMORNING SNACK: CARROT SHAKE (page 110). Add one tablespoon of granulated lecithin.

LUNCH: APPLE–CIDER VINEGAR DRINK (page 87), followed by SUPER SALAD (page 98) with FAT–LOSS DRESSING (pages 100 to 101) of choice. If you eat at a restaurant today, select one that has a salad bar and assemble a Super Salad from the raw vegetables and greens provided.

MIDAFTERNOON SNACK: Optional–CARROT SHAKE (page 110), or REJUVELAC (page 88), one cup.

DINNER: HIJIKI STIR–FRY (page 106); accompany with thick POTASSIUM BROTH (page 92), as much as you want.

EXERCISE: OXYGENATION COCKTAIL (page 82). YOGA SELF–MASSAGE (page 126) followed by thirty minutes of brisk walking.

EVENING ACTIVITY: (At home night): Begin preparations for CHAPARRAL DETOXIFYING BATH (page 157). Drink one cup of REJUVELAC (page 88). Add remainder to tonight's bath. HOT CASTOR OIL ABDOMINAL WRAP (page 186). While Castor Oil wrap is on, do THREE–PART BREATHING (page 137) and COMPLETE BREATH (page 138), and ALTERNATE–HEMISPHERE BREATHING (page 139). Follow with CHAPARRAL DETOXIFYING BATH.

TUESDAY: DAY 18

ON AWAKENING: One 8–ounce glass of HOT LEMON–WATER FLUSH (page 80); add one teaspoon honey with ROYAL JELLY (page 206). Prepare INNER BEAUTY HERBAL TEA (page 81); drink throughout the day between meals. Use INSPIROL (Cleansing Inhalant) (page 135).

MORNING CLEANSING: DRY BRUSH MASSAGE (page 144). Follow with hot shower, finishing with a one–minute cold splash.

BREAKFAST: CLEANSING WATERMELON BREAKFAST (page 92).

MIDMORNING SNACK: TAHINI SHAKE (page 110). Add one tablespoon of granulated lecithin.

LUNCH: APPLE–CIDER VINEGAR DRINK (page 87), followed by SUPER SALAD (page 98) with FAT–LOSS DRESSING (pages 100 to 101) of choice. If you eat at a restaurant today, select one that has a salad bar and assemble a Super Salad from the raw vegetables and greens provided.

MIDAFTERNOON SNACK: Optional–TAHINI SHAKE (page 110), or REJUVELAC (page 88), one cup.

DINNER: MISO SEA SOUP (page 107); steamed vegetables with WARM GARLIC DRESSING (page 104).

EXERCISE: OXYGENATION COCKTAIL (page 82). LYMPH– CLEAN

SING WARM–UP (page 118) followed by thirty minutes of brisk walking.

EVENING ACTIVITY: Drink one cup of REJUVELAC (page 88). Professional COLONIC IRRIGATION or CLEANSING ENEMA (page 188) accompanied by TUMMY MASSAGE (page 187). Follow with CLEOPATRA'S MILK BATH (page 158), using a batch of the barley water you made on Day 8.

WEDNESDAY: DAY 19

ON AWAKENING: One 8–ounce glass of HOT LEMON–WATER FLUSH (page 80); add one teaspoon honey with ROYAL JELLY (page 206). Prepare INNER BEAUTY HERBAL TEA (page 81); drink throughout the day between meals. Use INSPIROL (Cleansing Inhalant) (page 135). Prepare four cups of DIURETIC TEA (page 86); let steep all day for use in tonight's footbath.

MORNING CLEANSING: DRY BRUSH MASSAGE (page 144), followed by warm shower.

BREAKFAST: FRESH APPLE BREAKFAST (page 89).

MIDMORNING SNACK: Optional–MAPLE-NUT SHAKE (page 109), or REJUVELAC (page 88), one cup. Pour off today's REJUVELAC and prepare a batch for tomorrow. Have a protein drink in morning or afternoon only if you are hungry or need an energy boost.

LUNCH: Fish, chicken, or tofu with steamed or raw vegetables.

MIDAFTERNOON SNACK: Optional–MAPLE–NUT SHAKE (page 109), or REJUVELAC (page 88), one cup.

DINNER: Vegetable Bisque (pages 94 to 95) of choice.

EXERCISE: OXYGENATION COCKTAIL (page 82). DANCER'S WARM–UP (page 117), followed by thirty minutes of brisk walking.

EVENING ACTIVITY: Drink one cup of REJUVELAC (page 88). Add the remainder to tonight's footbath. CELLULITE SELF–EXAM (page 200), followed by CELLULITE MASSAGE (page 202) with CELLULITE MASSAGE OIL (page 200). Follow with "HOT FOOT" SOAK (page 162). Add REJUVELAC AND DIURETIC TEA you made this morning. Soak feet for twenty minutes.

THURSDAY: DAY 20

ON AWAKENING: One 8–ounce glass of HOT LEMON–WATER FLUSH (page 80); add one teaspoon honey with ROYAL JELLY (page 206). Prepare

INNER BEAUTY HERBAL TEA (page 81); drink throughout the day between meals. Use INSPIROL (Cleansing Inhalant) (page 135).

MORNING CLEANSING: DRY BRUSH MASSAGE (page 144). Follow with Alternating Hot and Cold Shower—begin with three to five minutes of hot water; switch to ten to fifteen seconds of cold water. Repeat three times, ending with cold water. Dry briskly with a coarse towel.

BREAKFAST: HEALING GRAPE BREAKFAST (page 89).

MIDMORNING SNACK: Optional—CARROT SHAKE (page 110) or REJU-VELAC (page 88), one cup. Pour off today's Rejuvelac and prepare a batch for tomorrow. Have a protein drink in morning or afternoon only if you are hungry or need an energy boost.

LUNCH: Fish, chicken or tofu with steamed or raw vegetables.

MIDAFTERNOON SNACK: Optional—CARROT SHAKE (page 110), or REJUVELAC (page 88), one cup.

DINNER: SQUASH BISQUE (page 94) and baked potato with GOLDEN GODDESS TOPPING (page 102).

EXERCISE: OXYGENATION COCKTAIL (page 82). WAKE–UP SHAKE–UP (page 116), followed by thirty minutes of brisk walking.

EVENING ACTIVITY: Drink one cup of REJUVELAC (page 88). Add the remainder to tonight's bath. YOGA REJUVENATION POSTURES (page 129), followed by BALLOON BREATHING (page 135). Follow with EVENING "YOUTH BATH" (page 154), or if you really cannot stand cold water tonight, a warm SEA–MINERAL BATH (page 154).

FRIDAY: DAY 21

ON AWAKENING: One 8–ounce glass of HOT LEMON–WATER FLUSH (page 80); add one teaspoon honey with ROYAL JELLY (page 206). Prepare INNER BEAUTY HERBAL TEA (page 81); drink throughout the day between meals. Use INSPIROL (Cleansing Inhalant) (page 135).

MORNING CLEANSING: MORNING COLD SPLASH AND RUB (page 154).

BREAKFAST: SLICED FRESH PINEAPPLE BREAKFAST (page 90).

MIDMORNING SNACK: Optional—TAHINI SHAKE (page 110), or REJU-VELAC (page 88), one cup. Pour off today's REJUVELAC and prepare a batch for tomorrow. Have a protein drink in morning or afternoon only if you are hungry or need an energy boost.

LUNCH: Fish, chicken, or tofu with steamed or raw vegetables.

MIDAFTERNOON SNACK: Optional—TAHINI SHAKE (page 110), or REJUVELAC (page 88), one cup.

DINNER: BEET BORSCHT (page 96) and steamed vegetables with CAR-ROT–LEEK PUREE (page 103).

EXERCISE: OXYGENATION COCKTAIL (page 82). LYMPH CLEAN-SING WARM–UP (page 118) followed by thirty minutes of brisk walking.

EVENING ACTIVITY: Drink one cup of REJUVELAC (page 88). Add the remainder to tonight's bath. Complete TOXICITY SYMPTOM CHECK-LIST (page 22). Review 21–DAY SPA GOALS CONTRACT (page 29). Apply HOT OLIVE–OIL REJUVENATING FACIAL (page 147). Leave olive oil on while taking OPTIMISM BATH (page 158). In bath, do WARM SOAK AND STROKE (page 177).

This week you have begun to integrate the wonderful cleansing and reju-venation activities, techniques and recipes into your everyday life to guarantee yourself many added years of vitality. Remember that you do not have to be on a special 21–Day Program to enjoy these self–nurturing activi-ties. For example, you can treat yourself to a massage with a footbath and herbal steam anytime you wish. As you encourage your body to build healthy, youthful cells to replace the old ones that are constantly dying and being eliminated, you turn back the clock on the aging process. Rejuvena-tion is truly the key to a more youthful and more satisfying life

WEEK THREE

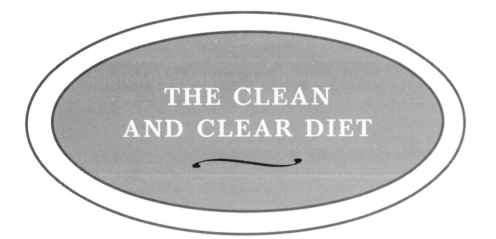

THE CLEAN
AND CLEAR DIET

*B*ack in my twenties, I was teaching in a public school, where I was encouraged to teach my students traditional dietary ideas about eating from the "four food groups" at every meal. Knowing how sluggish I felt when I followed the rules I was supposed to be teaching my students, and how wonderfully light and energetic I felt when I followed the principles of food-combining, I began to wonder if we were damaging our children by bringing them up with this misinformation about foods.

I have adapted the classic principles of food combining to create the Clean and Clear Diet that you will be following during most of the 21–Day Program. Each day's menu starts with a single raw-fruit breakfast, a protein–and–vegetable lunch, and a light dinner of vegetables and starch. You will be amazed at how energized you will feel as your body adjusts to this truly "balanced" diet. It may seem strange at first not to feel so full after meals. This is not because you won't be well nourished, but because you won't be so bloated. It may take a while for you to get used to this new sensation, as you begin to digest your foods in an easier way. As a side benefit, you will quickly notice a flatter tummy.

The Clean and Clear Diet is an absolutely essential preparation for the intensive cleansing your body will be undergoing in the second and third weeks of my program. This is why I want you to eat foods that are free of chemicals and contaminants, in combinations that are easy to digest. Such a diet will not add any more toxicity to your system, and it will minimize any cleansing reactions you may have later on. It is also the best diet for clearing your body of cellulite once and for all. In fact, the Clean and Clear Diet is so healthy and satisfying that it will change your eating habits permanently. It is a program you can stay on for the rest of your life!

HOW FOOD COMBINING WORKS

Although we eat for many different reasons, the ultimate physiological purpose of eating is to get nutrients into the blood so that we can build new cells to replace the ones that are constantly dying. Dead cells and other body wastes are removed from the body through the systems of elimination. When food is not properly digested, nutrients are not released, and it takes extra energy to remove the undigested waste from the system. This is why you may have noticed low energy and digestive discomfort when you eat heavy meals that are not properly combined.

The principles of food combining are based on an understanding of how the digestive process works. Different foods are digested in different ways, and they require different digestive juices to release the nutrients that can be used by your cells. Therefore, foods are eaten in combinations that promote efficient digestion and make the process extremely efficient. Conscious food combining has helped many people with long–standing digestion and elimination problems.

A good example is a client of mine named Marc, a Frenchman with a very successful import business. For fifteen years, he had gone from doctor to doctor to get help for his heartburn. Of course, he was used to eating the typical rich French foods. The doctors generally prescribed antacids, without giving him much advice on his diet.

When Marc came in to see me, his chief complaints were gas, bloating, and a feeling of burning and pressure after eating. I began with some intestinal cleansing for immediate relief. But mainly I worked with him on food–combining principles. By learning how to combine foods properly, Marc completely eliminated his heartburn and no longer needed antacids. It sounds amazingly simple, and it is. From time to time, however, Marc will eat a rich meal that combines a full spectrum of foods, but now he knows the reason when he has a feeling of burning afterward. He also knows that he can prepare his body for such occasions by taking digestive enzymes to support the digestive process. Marc is now in control of his body.

Heartburn and indigestion are only one kind of penalty you may pay for combining foods improperly. Constipation, flatulence, bloating, bad breath, cellulite, and overweight can all be signs that you are eating the wrong combinations of foods.

The Clean and Clear Diet follows five simple rules that work best for people whose main goals are relief from indigestion and gas, rejuvenation, weight loss, and renewed energy.

The Five Food-Combining Principles

1. Eat Fruit Alone. Every morning you will have a breakfast consisting of fresh fruit. This is a wonderful way to start the day, because fruit is a marvelous detoxifier. It has the highest water content of all foods, and travels through the body very quickly. Besides the nutrients that it provides, the fiber in fruit acts like a brush to keep the intestinal walls clean and clear. The soluble fibers in fruit also help to lower cholesterol in the blood.

Fruit is a very simple food. It contains sugars that are ready for the body to utilize, and provides its own enzymes, so it does not need much time to be digested in the stomach. Your goal is to pass fruit out of the stomach as quickly as possible, so that its nutrients will be absorbed rapidly through the walls of the small intestine and the colon. This is why you should not combine fruit with other foods, or have it too soon after eating protein or starch. If you do, the sugar in the fruit will ferment in the stomach, causing bloating and gas pain.

Generally, fruits may be combined with each other, but melons should be eaten alone, because they are made up almost entirely of water and need very little time to digest. Combining melon with another kind of fruit will cause it to be held up in the stomach, and it will begin to ferment.

After eating fruit, allow at least two hours before eating any other kind of food. Morning is the best time to eat fruit, because then you can be certain other foods have already left the stomach. Please do not eat fruit for dessert after a meal. It will be held up in your stomach by the other foods, causing it to ferment.

You may wonder why I recommend a light fruit breakfast, when, traditionally, dietitians advise us to eat a hearty breakfast consisting of foods from all four food groups. Your body really does not need much food in the morning, because it is still utilizing the nutrients from the food you ate the night before. Fruit helps to raise your blood sugar and cleanse the wastes from your system.

If you find this light breakfast is not enough for you, please honor that message from yourself, as there are several metabolic types of people. We all differ slightly in our nutrient needs. This is why I recommend the protein drink two hours after the fruit breakfast for some of you.

2. Do Not Combine Protein with Starch. Protein foods and starchy foods require different digestive juices in order to be properly broken down and used by the body. The digestion of starches begins in the mouth with the enzyme ptyalin, which is contained in your saliva. Proteins are mainly broken down in the stomach, by hydrochloric acid and the protein-splitting enzyme pepsin. Please avoid the traditional American dinner of meat and potatoes, or meat and other starches, as well as sandwiches containing cheese, meats, eggs, or other proteins. When you think about how regularly we consume these combinations, it is no wonder that indigestion remedies are among the best–selling over–the–counter medicines in this country!

When protein and starch are eaten together, ptyalin is not effectively produced in the saliva, and so the starch is not predigested in the mouth. It enters the stomach and begins to ferment, producing gas. To make matters worse, protein needs to be digested in an acid environment and starch in an alkaline environment. So, when starches and proteins are combined, the acid and alkaline digestive juices neutralize each other! All this decaying food is held up in the stomach, causing gas and discomfort. More important, the nutrients you need to rejuvenate and replenish your cells are destroyed in the decaying and fermenting process. This dietary cycle can eventually lead to premature aging and illness.

When I speak of protein foods, I am referring mainly to animal proteins. Some plant foods, such as beans, contain natural combinations of starches and proteins. If these foods are eaten alone, the body is able to digest them properly by releasing the proper digestive juices in the proper sequence. Even so, some people do feel uncomfortable after eating beans.

3. Protein with Vegetables is Okay. Your midday meals in the first week of the program will consist of a protein food–fish or chicken or tofu–and non-starch vegetables. Vegetables are high in water content and are relatively easy to digest. They can be broken down in either an acid or alkaline environment. And so they can be combined with proteins as well as with starches. The enzymes in the vegetables actually enhance the digestion of protein. The fiber contained in vegetables helps to move the non–fiber protein foods rapidly through the intestines.

4. Starches with Vegetables Are Okay, Too. Since vegetables do not require their own specific digestive juices, they can be digested in the alkaline environment required by starches. Your evening meal each day in Week 1 will be based on vegetables and starchy foods. You will feel and see the benefits right away when you begin to eat your lighter meal in the evening rather than at lunchtime. Your body will respond by speedily digesting your dinner while you sleep. By morning, your body will be clean and clear again, ready for its final flushing with a fruit breakfast.

5. Do Not Drink with Meals. If you drink water, tea or any other beverage along with your meal, you dilute the digestive juices that are needed to break down your food, preventing it from being properly digested. The best time to drink fluids is between meals–at least one–half hour before or two hours after. Remember, you will be drinking at least eight full glasses of water each day, including herbal tea and other rehydrating drinks I will recommend. If you are eating fruits and vegetables, which are high in water content, or beans and grains that are prepared with water, then the food itself will provide plenty of fluid, and you should not feel thirsty after your meal. If you do find that you are thirsty after eating, you may be consuming too much salt.

FOOD COMBINING FOR YOUR BUSY LIFESTYLE

Do you ever experience a midafternoon slump, when you just seem to run out of energy? These low points may be caused by a drop in your blood-sugar level. Part of the reason why you will be eating protein at lunchtime is to help boost your blood–sugar level and keep you on an even keel throughout the afternoon.

If your busy schedule requires that you eat your fruit breakfast very early in the morning, and then you have a late lunch, you may notice that you get lightheaded or irritable sometime in the midmorning. This may also happen if you are accustomed to having a heavier breakfast. For those who need a midmorning boost, I have provided recipes for protein drinks, beginning on page 107. You can make your protein drink in the morning and take it with you in a thermos to work. Always be sure to wait two hours after eating your fruit breakfast before you consume the protein drink, to allow time for the fruit to leave your stomach. (Because you will have protein at lunch, the timing between your midmorning protein drink and your lunch is not as critical.)

In the midafternoon, if you feel your energy begin to flag again, have some fresh carrot juice. Carrot juice is very high in natural sugar, so it will raise your blood sugar and help control your craving for sweets. Fresh carrot juice is available at some supermarkets and at juice bars and health–food stores everywhere. If necessary, stock up on fresh carrot juice, and bring it with you to work.

Allowing for variations in routine, your daily meal schedule will look something like this:

> Between 6:00 and 10:00 A.M.: Breakfast
> Between 12:00 and 3:00 P.M.: Lunch
> Between 5:00 and 8:00 P.M. : Dinner

These meal periods allow the ideal time for the food to pass out of the stomach before you eat different foods at your next meal.

You can dine out in restaurants the entire time on the Clean and Clear Diet, if you wish. Using the simple rules of food combining, you can always choose the proper meals in a restaurant.

Whenever you eat out, you need to make a choice. You are going to have either a protein meal, or a starch meal. If you choose a protein meal, then you must exclude starch, and that means excluding bread! Many people find it helpful to ask the waiter not to bring bread to the table. If you are ordering fish or chicken–which is generally served with rice, pasta, or potatoes–ask your waiter to leave off the starch and bring extra vegetables instead. I have never found a restaurant that was not willing to do that. If you choose a starch meal, such as a pasta dish, be sure that it does not include protein or dairy products in the sauce. You might want to ask for a simple tomato sauce or an olive oil and garlic sauce. Often you will not find a vegetable main dish on the menu, but more and more restaurants will gladly prepare a plate of steamed or sauteed vegetables with a side order of rice, a baked potato, or pasta.

If you eat at a salad bar, remember that you must apply the rules of food combining just as at any other restaurant. Before you make any selections, you must choose between a protein meal and a starch meal. Help yourself to plenty of vegetables, but do not combine a high–protein food such as garbanzo beans with starch crackers or rolls. Stay away from cheeses and other dairy products entirely, and remember not to combine fruits with other foods.

Certain foods in restaurants should be avoided. Prepared salad dressings are often loaded with fats, salt, and preservatives. If you have not brought your own salad dressing with you, ask for olive oil and fresh lemon. Also be careful about ordering soups in restaurants, because they are often loaded with salt and cream. Salt holds fluid in the tissues, and you are trying to continually flush the fluids out of your tissues. Cutting down on your salt consumption helps to speed this process.

Did you know that airlines offer a wide variety of special–order meals, such as fresh fruit plates or vegetable plates? Think ahead, and at the time that you make your reservation, request a special vegetarian meal or some other selection that allows you to follow your food–combining rules.

One of my clients, Amy, is a bank manager who had been eating an unhealthy junk–food diet to comfort herself because of emotional problems connected with a failing relationship. When she started her cleansing program, her abdomen was extremely distended, her skin had a yellowish tinge, and she had a strong body odor. Her eyes and her whole body were puffy from water retention. As she changed her diet and started to clean out her system, her skin color changed noticeably. After a couple of months on my program, she had rosy cheeks again, and she even began to change the color scheme of her wardrobe and makeup because her complexion had improved so much. She had previously been very embarrassed about her offensive body odor and had been using a lot of deodorant and perfume to conceal it. As she began to detoxify, her natural scent became fresh and clean.

Although Amy's original purpose had been to clean the toxins out of her system, she also experienced remarkable weight loss. During the second week of the program, she began to notice that she was urinating a great deal and was starting to lose the bloated feeling that had accompanied the water retention. Moreover, as she eliminated the foods from her diet that had been so difficult for her body to digest, her energy began to come back, and she wanted to resume regular exercise. As she stepped up her exercise, of course, she lost more weight.

Amy became a great proponent of food combining. Her management job required her to eat out a lot. She noticed that if she was careful about food combining, she would have high energy all day. If she broke her food combining rules, she would feel lethargic and bloated.

So many of us have been on and off diets all our lives. We binge, binge, binge, then starve, starve, starve. Of course, this never works. By following the simple principles of the Clean and Clear Diet, you can eat delicious food throughout the day and still lose weight. Once your body starts getting rid of the waste that has been clogging your systems of elimination, you will have increased energy, your skin will take on a more youthful appearance and your craving for junk foods will be replaced by a genuine desire to eat clean, healthy foods.

CLEAN AND CLEAR FOODS

The Clean and Clear Diet features simple, fresh, organically raised foods. Make no mistake about it; clean foods are delicious. In the Body–Smart Recipes on pages 79 through 110), I'm going to show you how to prepare meals that are combined properly, and that have no junk in them at all—no

---

COOKBOOKS THAT SUPPORT THE CLEAN AND CLEAR PROGRAM

Steam Cuisine *by Annette Annechild and Laura Johnson (Macmillan)*

The Book of Whole Meals *by Annemarie Colbin (Ballantine)*

California Sea Food Cookbook *by Isaac Cronin, Jay Harlow, and Paul Johnson (Aris)*

Natural Foods Cookbook *by Mary Estella (Japan Publications USA)*

Ten Talents Vegetarian Natural Foods Cookbook *by Frank and Rosalie Hurd (Ten Talents)*

McDougall Health Supporting Cookbook *Vols. I and II, by Mary A. McDougall (New Century)*

Grain Gastronomy *by Janet Fletcher (Aris)*

preservatives, no additives, no heavy fats, no chemicals. I will introduce some special recipes that will help to stimulate your systems of elimination and nourish every cell in your body to make you feel and look lighter, more youthful, and more energetic.

Fruits and Vegetables

At the very heart of the Clean and Clear Diet are fresh fruits and vegetables. Our bodies are at least 70 percent water, and since fruits and vegetables also are very high in water, they are most perfectly suited to our body composition. The water contained in fruits and vegetables is important for nourishing and cleansing. Water carries the rich cargo of nutrients into the intestines, where they are rapidly absorbed. The water then flushes away the wastes. Of course, you should use organic fruits and vegetables. If you are not able to get organic produce, use the food–cleansing soak described on page 88 .

Although I recommend that many vegetables be eaten raw, as in salads, you will also be eating cooked vegetables. The best cooking methods are those in which the vegetables are cooked the least, such as steaming, sauteing in a wok, or microwave cooking. There are many good natural–foods cookbooks that provide instructions on these cooking methods.

Vegetables need not be eaten plain to be healthy. The recipes for nourishing Clean and Clear Toppings, beginning on page 102, are a delicious accompaniment for cooked vegetables. Some of these toppings use vegetables as a base and are also suitable for use on starchy foods or protein dishes. Other are based on proteins and make a complete meal with raw or cooked vegetables.

I am emphasizing vegetables in the Clean and Clear Diet because we are focusing on mineralizing the system. Many of the recipes in this book—the broths, teas, protein drinks, and vegetable soups—are extremely high in minerals. Because our soil is so depleted today, it is not necessarily true that people can get all the nutrients they need from their food. This is why I will recommend a program of nutritional supplements later in this chapter on page 72.

An excellent way to get minerals into your body is to make mineral–rich vegetable soups. Long a mainstay of the biological clinics in Europe, vegetable broths are very beneficial for anyone on a cleansing, fasting, and alkalinizing program. On page 92 I provide you with the recipe for Potassium Broth, a base for delicious, clean vegetable soups and bisques that provide nutrients your body needs to promote cleansing and rejuvenation.

Another source of abundant minerals is sea vegetables. Edible seaweeds have long been a regular part of the diet of coastal peoples such as the Japanese, the Pacific Islanders, and the Irish. Extremely rich in iodine and other minerals, sea vegetables are a very important food for beautiful hair, skin, and nails, and for healthy bones and teeth. The iodine in sea vegetables stimulates the thyroid gland, ensuring proper metabolism and promoting a healthy reproductive system. While you may have only eaten seaweed before as a wrapping for sushi, during the vegetarian phase of this program you will enjoy the Hijiki Stir–Fry on page 106. You may also add small amounts of dried seaweed to any soup for a flavorful dash of concentrated sea minerals.

Miracle Foods

Some foods provide such marvelous combination of taste, nutrition, and health benefits that they truly deserve to be called miracle foods. They are so beneficial that I recommend that you consume them every day during your three–week program.

Garlic and Onions Garlic has long been valued for its healing properties. In World War II, it was used against typhus and dysentery, and its germ–killing and immune–strengthening actions have been widely documented by modern researchers. Garlic is very helpful against yeast and fungus infections. The active ingredient in garlic is the volatile oil allicin, which gives garlic its unmistakable smell, and which is able to kill harmful bacteria without hurting your body's naturally friendly bacteria.

Garlic is rich in selenium, a powerful anti–aging nutrient, and has been shown to be helpful in controlling high blood pressure, heart disease, intestinal problems, liver disorders, and sinus conditions. Recent medical research has shown that garlic is very powerful in reducing cholesterol and triglyceride levels in the blood. By reducing the stickiness of platelets, it prevents blood from clotting, thereby helping to protect against heart attacks. As a demonstration of garlic's life–extending powers, a study in India of people over one hundred years old found that the only common factor they shared was that they all consumed large quantities of this aromatic bulb.

Garlic is best eaten raw. You can dice or crush it and add it to vegetable salad, soup, or any cooked dish. Raw garlic produces a stronger odor than cooked garlic. Chewing some fresh parsley will help to mask the garlic odor on your breath. Garlic capsules are also available, but read the labeling to make sure that they contain the active ingredient allicin.

Onions belong to the same plant family as garlic, and like garlic, onions help to bring down cholesterol levels and to prevent the clumping together of platelets. These two vegetables, especially eaten together raw, help to prevent the accumulation of unwelcome fats in the arteries that can lead to heart attacks and strokes.

Lecithin A derivative of soybeans, lecithin can be purchased as a supplement in granular form at health food stores. Lecithin contains acetylcholine, which helps to remove lactic–acid wastes from the body, making the joints and muscles more flexible. It flushes fat out of the liver and prevents its accumulation in the bloodstream. Lecithin washes wastes away from the nerve cells and improves the reflexes.

Sprouts Sprouted seeds, whole grains, and legumes are among the healthiest foods you can eat. They are a perfect example of a living food that carries nutrients in the most beneficial form directly to your cells.

The sprouting of seeds for food was recorded in China as far back as 3000 B.C. Sprouts are extremely high in the purest forms of protein, and they contain cholesterol–reducing lecithin. Sprouts are rich in enzymes that trigger increased activity in your digestive system. Sprouts are also full of vitamins and minerals, and are extremely low in calories.

The produce sections of supermarkets and health–food stores will often have different kinds of sprouts available. However, in places where it may be difficult to get fresh or organically grown food, growing your own sprouts at home is a simple way to guarantee a source of clean, living food.

Alfalfa seeds are the easiest to begin with, but you can use other seeds or grains such as lentils, mung beans, rye, yellow soy, wheat, sunflower, and radish.

Sprouting Seeds At Home

Try to find alfalfa seeds prepared especially for sprouting. These are becoming increasingly common in health–food stores. Otherwise, buy food–quality seeds.

Place two tablespoons of alfalfa seeds in a one–quart glass jar with a screened lid. These jars are generally sold in health–food stores and hardware stores. Fill the jar with purified water and cap it. Let the seeds soak overnight. Pour the water off in the morning. Add fresh purified water and pour it off again to rinse the seeds.

Place the jar upside down and slightly tilted, so it can drain. Keep it in a dark place or cover with a towel. Rinse the seeds twice a day, in the morning before you leave for work and in the evening when you get home, by filling the jar with water through the screened lid, then pouring it out. After two or three days, the sprouts will be ready for eating.

You can use this same procedure for sprouting other seeds and grains. However, use only one tablespoon of the larger seeds, such as sunflower seeds, in a quart–sized jar.

The Super Salad on page 98 is a great way of making sure you get all the miracle foods I have discussed, as well as other nutritious ingredients.

Whole Grains

Whole, unprocessed grains are an excellent choice for your starchy meals. They contain important nutrients that processing has removed from much of the food in the American diet, such as B vitamins, vitamin E, and bran fiber that helps to cleanse the walls of your intestines.

While you are practicing proper food combining on the Clean and Clear Diet, you have an excellent opportunity to experiment with some new grains. Remember, however, that grains are starchy foods, and should not be combined with animal protein.

Many grain cookbooks are now appearing in bookstores, as more and more people recognize the benefits of these wholesome foods. There are four grains that I find to be especially healthful and delicious.

Buckwheat Buckwheat is the staple grain in the USSR, where it is made into a porridge call kasha. Soviet scientists attribute the life–extending and rejuvenating properties of buckwheat to the fact that it contains rutin, a bioflavonoid, which helps to keep blood pressure down. Buckwheat contains complete, high quality vegetable proteins and many vitamins, and is especially rich in the minerals manganese, magnesium, and potassium. Because the proteins in buckwheat are a natural component of the grain, your digestive system supplies the proper enzymes in the right order to make use of this vegetable protein, as long as it is not improperly combined with other proteins, such as meats.

MILLET The staple grain throughout much of the Near and Far East and Africa, millet has been eaten by human beings longer than any other grain. The ancient Greeks and before them the Egyptians recognized its high nutritional value. Millet is a complete protein food, containing all the essential amino acids, and is thus comparable to meat or milk in its protein value. It is extremely rich in vitamins and minerals, especially calcium, magnesium, and trace elements such as molybdenum. It alkalinizes the system, unlike most grains, and hence is nonfattening since alkalis tend to dissolve fat and counteract its accumulation in the body. Millet is also extremely tasty.

QUINOA Native to the Andes Mountains, quinoa (pronounced keen–wa) has been a staple food for thousands of years. Health–conscious American visitors, impressed by the extremely high nutritional value of quinoa, have recently brought this grain back to the United States, and are now cultivating it in the Colorado Rockies. You can find it in many health–food stores, along with recipes for preparing it. Quinoa has a higher protein content that any other grain, and has an interesting, nut like flavor. It is more expensive than other grains, because it is still relatively rare.

BARLEY Praised for its strengthening and invigorating properties, barley was eaten by the Roman gladiators and is used extensively today in many parts of the world, particularly the Middle East. Its fiber, known as beta glucans and also found in oats, helps to lower blood cholesterol, prevent constipation, and improve bowel function in general. Barley is a great nourisher of the nerve cells and helps to calcify the bones. The most beneficial forms of barley are the least processed, such as whole–grain barley, barley grits, and barley flakes, all available in health–food stores. Barley is also the base for Rejuvelac, a fermented beauty drink that I introduce on page 88.

Protein Foods

Even our more conservative dietary establishment has recognized that Americans eat much more protein than their bodies require. Too much protein in the diet creates toxic nitrogen by–products that place an extra burden on the kidneys. Studies also show that populations that eat high animal–protein diets run a greatly increased risk of developing cancer.

The Clean and Clear Diet provides a fully adequate supply of protein every day, although you may be eating less protein than you are accustomed to. As a result, you may notice a lighter feeling and an overall improvement in your digestion. In particular, I want to emphasize reducing your consumption of animal protein. I do not recommend red meats during the 21–Day Program, so when you do buy flesh foods, please select chicken or fish. Range–fed chicken is the best choice for chicken, and deep–water ocean fish come from a less polluted part of the ocean. For your fish or chicken meals, select a simple cooking method such as broiling, grilling, or steaming.

Avoid cooking methods that use fats. (After you have finished your 21–Day Program you may occasionally want to add red meat to your diet. Please be sure to select organically raised beef or lamb in order to avoid ingesting the hormones fed to mass–produced animals.)

Another option for your protein meals is tofu, which is made from soy-beans. The cookbooks listed in this chapter on page 66 contain recipes for tofu main dishes. On pages 104 through 105, I have given some recipes for tofu toppings that make a satisfying protein accompaniment to raw or cooked vegetables.

As you select your protein meals, try to select a different source of protein every day. You can consider each kind of fish as a different type of protein. Rotate your selections so that you are not eating the same protein more than once every four days. This will reduce the stress on your digestive system.

I advocate a restriction of dairy products on the Clean and Clear Diet. During the three–week program, you should consume no milk and no cheese at all. Many people have a hard time digesting milk, while cheese congests the system and dehydrates the body, which makes is one of the most constipating foods. Later on, when you have completed the program, you should consider cheese as an infrequent high–fat treat, not a dietary staple.

Except for a small amount of butter, the only other dairy food I would recommend at all is yogurt. Yogurt is easier to assimilate than other dairy products, because the fermentation process has broken down the milk sugar. I suggest that you not eat yogurt too often–no more than every fourth day. For those who enjoy an occasional yogurt dish, I have given you a recipe for a yogurt topping on page 104, and for a yogurt–enriched beet borscht on page 96.

Many people are reluctant to cut down on their intake of dairy products because they are afraid they will not get enough calcium. There are many sources of calcium besides dairy products, including raw sesame seeds, raw nuts, corn tortillas, leafy greens such as kale, broccoli, mustard, watercress and parsley, and sea vegetables, especially dulse and kelp. Also, most people benefit from calcium supplements, no matter what foods they eat.

Nuts and seeds are alternative sources of protein that can be made into satisfying and nourishing protein drinks. Such drinks are an important part of your three–week program. There are several recipes on pages 107 to 110.

Fats

Many people believe that if you want to lose weight and prevent heart disease, you cannot eat any fat at all. The truth is that there are some good fats that are essential to your health and beauty. To maximize your health, prevent the effects of aging, and flush the fat out of your body, you need a daily supply of these good fats, known as Omega–3 and Omega–6 oils, or EPAs and GLAs.

Often my clients come to me for help after years of intermittently starving their bodies on low–calorie, very low–fat diets. Among their complaints,

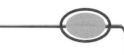

they mention dry hair and skin, weak and brittle nails, as well as problems of elimination. By adding the essential GLA and EPA oils to their diet, we are able to reverse these problems to restore healthy, glowing skin, shiny hair, and strong nails.

GLAs and EPAs are necessary for the manufacture of prostaglandin, hormone-like compounds that regulate all your bodily functions at the molecular level. Every cell in your body needs a daily supply of these essential fats in order to produce these all-important prostaglandin.

The Omega-3 fats, or EPAs, are polyunsaturated oils whose richest source is oily cold-water fish such as herring, salmon, mackerel, cod, sardines, rainbow trout, and halibut. It is the EPA in the diet of Eskimos that prevents them from having heart disease, despite a diet composed almost entirely of animal protein and fat. Other societies that consume large quantities of fish have also been found to have a low incidence of heart disease, confirming the protective value of the EPAs.

EPA makes the blood platelets less sticky, helping the blood to flow more freely and preventing clots in the heart and blood vessels. It helps to bring down blood-fat levels, and may also help reduce the stiffness and aching of arthritis. You can supply some of your EPA requirement by eating cold-water fish two or three times a week. EPA is also available in supplement form at pharmacies and health-food stores.

The Omega-6 polyunsaturated oils, or GLAs, are even more important than the EPAs for protecting the heart and cardiovascular system, the immune system, and the skin. GLAs help flush fats out of the body, and when GLA and EPA are taken together, the production of health-promoting prostaglandin is maximized.

Unrefined vegetable oils, especially safflower oil, contain the raw material for the GLA that the body needs. Evening-primrose and borage oils are naturally high in GLA, and other high GLA oils include sunflower, corn, soy, and sesame. Always be sure when you buy safflower or other high-GLA oil that it is cold-pressed and unrefined.

On the Clean and Clear Diet, I recommend that you use two tablespoons of safflower oil each day, to ensure that you get the required amount of fat-flushing GLAs. The salad dressings beginning on page 100 are based on safflower and sesame oil, both excellent sources of GLAs. Use these dressings regularly on your salads to promote healthy hair, skin, and nails, and provide the anti-aging benefits of a clean and clear circulatory and cardiovascular system.

Heat changes polyunsaturated oils, creating free radicals—substances that age your body prematurely. For this reason, when you use oil for cooking, never use safflower oil. Use olive oil instead, since it can stand higher temperatures. Recent research has shown that olive oil in the diet selectively reduces levels of LDL, the dangerous form of blood cholesterol, while keeping the beneficial form, or HDL, intact. This may explain why Mediterranean peoples such as the Greeks and Italians, who use olive oil as a staple in their diet, have half the mortality rate from heart disease than

Americans do. Olive oil contains mono–unsaturated fat, as do avocados and nuts. Another recently discovered mono–unsaturated oil is canola oil, which can also be used in cooking. While you should still be careful not to consume too much fat, you may enjoy these delicious foods in moderation without fear of damaging your heart and arteries.

For cooking, you may also use a little butter, but definitely avoid margarine because it is made of oils that have been chemically altered through hydrogenation, producing toxic substances.

Supplements

During the 21–Day Program, I would like you to fortify yourself with the extra protection of a simple combination of supplements. While I certainly believe that you should get as much nutrition as possible from your food, it is a fact of modern life that there are some nutrients that you are not going to be able to get enough of. Also, until you have completed this cleansing program, it is likely that you are not absorbing all the nutrients that you are eating, since your digestive system is probably not yet functioning up to par. A goal of this program is to make your absorption of nutrients more efficient, but in the meantime I recommend the following supplementation.

First of all, take a good high–potency multivitamin supplement each day. It is also a good idea to take an extra vitamin E plus selenium, and a calcium/magnesium supplement.

Always take your supplements with meals. If you take your supplements on an empty stomach, or wash them down with only water or juice, chances are that they will not be absorbed and used very efficiently by your body. Taking your supplements with food also prevents the possibility of stomach upset.

Make sure you are getting your daily requirement of beneficial GLA and EPA oil. The safflower oil in your salad dressing every day will help cover your need for GLA. You can also take safflower–oil capsules. To provide your EPA, you can supplement the fish in your diet by taking EPA capsules, derived from fish oil. Both supplements are available in health–food stores.

I also recommend that you use liquid minerals. This is an extract of key minerals that are suspended in liquid form in an ionic state.

BODY INTELLIGENCE: FOOD SENSITIVITIES AND YOUR OPTIMAL DIET

Do you have annoying little symptoms that always seem to be there, that you have accepted as "normal" for you? You may have constantly clogged sinuses, or mood swings, or a rapid heartbeat or tired feeling sometimes after eating. You may dismiss these problems by saying, "That's just the way I am; I have to live with it." But the real problem may be food sensitivities. One of the benefits of the light diet and the thorough cleansing of my Cleansing and Rejuvenation Program is that it eliminates many of the foods to which people are often sensitive. Essentially, I am helping you to do what allergy doctors do–to give your immune system a rest and cleanse your body before you begin to reintroduce foods to which you may be sensitive.

PROBLEM FOODS AND THEIR SYMPTOMS

While food sensitivities can produce a wide and often unpredictable range of symptoms in different people, some foods seem to show reaction patterns in the symptoms they provoke. The following are some of the common patterns that have been observed:

Milk and Dairy Products, Including Cheese

Respiratory symptoms such as runny nose, sinus problems, asthma; ear infections; gastrointestinal symptoms such as gas, cramps, bloating, diarrhea, constipation.

Wheat

Mental and behavioral problems; water retention.

Nightshade Foods (potato, tomato, eggplant, bell peppers)

Arthritis and joint pain; headache.

Citrus Fruits (orange, lemon, grapefruit, angerine)

Hives, wheezing, headache.

Caffeine (coffee, cocoa, chocolate, cola drinks)

Headache, heart palpitations.

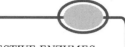

The most common problem foods are dairy products and wheat; some others include corn, eggs, soy products, shellfish, and yeast. Hopefully, as you complete the cleansing phase of the program and return to the Clean and Clear Diet, you will continue to avoid dairy products and wheat, the two most common offenders. In fact, part of the reason why you feel so wonderful during the 21–Day Program may be that you are no longer experiencing uncomfortable symptoms that food sensitivities may have caused in the past. Food sensitivities can cause a tremendously wide range of symptoms, including skin rashes, gastrointestinal problems, respiratory symptoms, fluctuations in blood sugar, swollen and painful joints, and food cravings.

I am sure that you will lose weight on this program. Part of this weight loss may be the result of giving up foods to which you are sensitive. Although no one seems to understand it completely, I believe that much excess weight is caused by the body retaining fluid in its tissues to protect itself against foods to which it is sensitive. When you eliminate these substances from your diet, the fluid is flushed out of the tissues. This is why you can lose weight so rapidly on a highly restricted diet. Of course, if you go back to eating the same foods again, you will put the weight right back on, as your body retains fluid to protect itself.

I know this is true from personal experience. I once lost fifteen pounds in three weeks, and the only change I had made in my diet was to give up eating wheat entirely, including all breads, pastas, and muffins. The weight just fell away as my kidneys eliminated the excess water from my system. Such experiences have shown me that wheat is a problem food for me. I also know that since childhood wheat bread has been the food I have turned to for comfort when I am upset. I am not alone in having this problem with bread and other wheat products. In fact, I consider bread the number–one enemy for anyone who has problems with weight control, constipation, and cellulite!

Besides the physical reactions that food sensitivities can cause, you may be surprised to learn that they can have very profound psychological effects. Wheat products are particularly troublesome in this regard. Research in the 1940's showed that many hospitalized schizophrenic patients' symptoms were relieved when they stopped eating wheat and related grain products. If they ate a little bread, they would reexperience their mental symptoms once again. Food sensitivities are now recognized as a very important factor in all sorts of mental and behavioral problems. Several years ago, Dr. Ben Feingold created a sensation when he developed the so–called Feingold diet, which eliminates foods to which children are often sensitive. On this diet, many children with hyperkinetic behavior problems settle down and improve markedly. Correctional and probation officers have found that special restricted diets can help to control criminal behavior, and even some marriage counselors are now taking a look at nutritional factors in dealing with family discord.

After you have finished the 21–Day Program, as you return to eating a full range of foods, you can experiment cautiously to try to discover your food sensitivities. If you suspect that your are sensitive to a certain food, eat quite a bit of it during one day—for example, eat some at breakfast and again

DIGESTIVE ENZYMES: A "FORGIVENESS FACTOR" IN YOUR DIET

When you make an educated choice to miscombine foods, or when you overindulge in your favorite delicacy, help your digestive system by taking a high–quality, multi–phase digestive enzyme.

Multi–phase enzyme supplements have two stages. They release hydrochloric acid and acidic enzymes in the stomach, and then, when they reach the small intestine, they release other alkaline enzymes needed for this basic environment. Take digestive enzymes before you eat a heavy meal to prevent bloating hours afterward. Most people are especially deficient in enzymes that produce hydrochloric acid.

Influenced by television advertising, people generally believe their digestive upset is caused by too much stomach acid, and so they take antacids to ease their symptoms. These remedies slow down or stop the digestive process without solving the underlying problems. Digestive enzymes can help you to derive maximum benefit from your food. You can find a variety of digestive enzymes in most health–food stores.

at lunch—and then take note of your reactions. Pay attention not only to physical symptoms such as digestive upset or headache, but also to any mental or emotional changes—whether you get sleepy, or your energy drops, or you become irritable. These reactions can all be signs that you are sensitive to the food in question. Be careful with these experiments. Now that your body has been cleaned out, you no longer have the mucoid coating in your intestines that protected you against these offending substances (as well as interfering with the absorption of essential nutrients), so the reactions that you experience may be more pronounced than they were in the past.

If you do discover a food to which you are sensitive, that does not necessarily mean that you can never eat it again. You simply do not want to expose your body to too much of it, or too often. Medical allergists generally recommend that once you have stayed away from a problem food for some time, you can begin to add it back into your diet as long as you only eat it once every four days. This is the so-called rotation diet, which is based on the principle of allowing your body to rest after exposure to a food to which you may be sensitive. In my practice, I have observed that it works better to eat suspect foods no more than once a week. Also, if there are two foods that you know you are sensitive to—for example, dairy and wheat—try not to eat them together, so that you do not place an added burden on your body.

As you return to a regular diet, it is still best to rotate even the foods to which you are not sensitive, especially proteins, which are the hardest to digest. It is better to eat a different protein food every day, and not to repeat the same protein more than once every four days. Generally, for foods that you are not sensitive to, repeating them no more than once every four days will avoid any possible problems. This principle of food rotation not only protects your immune system by allowing it to rest from food sensitivity reactions, but it also ensures that you receive the full spectrum of vitamins, minerals, and amino acids that are provided in perfect balance when you eat from all the foods in nature.

There will be times in the future when you cannot observe the food-rotation principle, or you will miscombine foods, or eat too much protein. An excellent aid at such times is a good digestive enzyme. After you have completed your At-Home Program, you may also experiment with some variations in the food-combining rules that I introduced earlier in this chapter. One variation is to combine acid fruits such as pineapple, berries, or oranges with light nut and seed proteins. Once your digestive system has been cleansed and healed by following the 21-Day Program, you can try making a smoothie using a protein drink base with strawberries, pineapple, or orange juice added. You can also make a fruit salad that combines acid fruits with nuts and seeds. Because papaya contains a great many enzymes, many people can combine papaya with proteins of all kinds without experiencing bloating. Pay attention to your physical reactions to determine whether these combinations work for you.

Many allergy-oriented health professionals believe that people crave the very foods to which they are allergic. I do not necessarily agree with this point of view. I think that your body has an innate, built-in wisdom, and that if you crave something, what you crave is not necessarily harmful for you.

Rather, I believe the craving is an indication that your body needs some particular kind of nutrient to restore its natural balance.

Cravings for sweets are a good example of this "body intelligence." Most people with whom I work in my practice, particularly women, tend to have sweet cravings, especially before their menstrual period. These cravings are not necessarily a sign of poor self–control; they are often a signal that something is lacking in the diet. I generally find that my clients' sweet cravings are a sign that they need more protein, especially early in the day. When my clients balance out their diets and find the one that is best for them, then sweet cravings usually go away.

Many people, for excellent philosophical reasons, try to follow a pure vegetarian diet, or a raw–foods diet, and find that it simply does not work for them. Their philosophical commitment may prevent them from noticing the warning signs, such as sweet or starch cravings, that their bodies need certain foods that they are not getting.

We are all looking for the diet that is best for our physical and mental well–being. We are also all unique individuals, and what is best for one person may not be best for another. Many health professionals, after extensive experimentation on themselves, become very tuned in to their own bodies. They proceed to write a book about having found the perfect diet, and act as though what they have discovered is best for everyone. I do not want to do that with you; that is why I keep asking you to notice how you feel. After cleansing your body, you will be much more sensitive to the personal effect of various foods. Pay particular attention as you add foods back to your diet, and continue to be vigilant after you complete this program. You are the one who can best recognize the signs that something is not right.

By becoming sensitive to your body's own needs, you will learn to make proper adjustments in your diet. You will know when you need an extra protein drink to pick up your energy or balance your nutrient intake, use digestive enzymes when you miscombine foods or eat too much protein, and use natural aids such as Rejuvelac on page 88 or the Apple–Cider Vinegar Drink on page 87, to enhance the work of your digestive system.

If you have a severe problem with food sensitivities or with finding the right balance of foods for you, you may want to seek guidance from a nutritionally oriented holistic physician. The Referral Guide to Holistic Practitioners on page 230 lists referral sources for physicians who have expertise in identifying food sensitivities and nutritional needs. If you do not have serious problems, you can use the tips I have provided in this chapter to experiment on your own, abstaining from the foods you suspect and then noticing what happens when you reintroduce them.

NOURISHING YOUR WHOLE SELF

Everyone knows that your emotions have great impact on the efficiency of your digestive processes. The best way to eat is in pleasant, calm surroundings. Put yourself in a relaxed mood, with no distractions such as television or a book. Before you begin eating, take a few deep breaths to calm and center yourself. You can then truly appreciate your meal. Eating your food consciously not only helps digestion, but it also prevents overeating, since you taste and appreciate every bite.

From childhood on, our social lives tend to center almost entirely around food. When Grandmother comes to visit, she brings the kids cookies; when you are good, you are rewarded with an ice–cream cone; when you go out on a date, you often go to a nice restaurant. Under these circumstances, it is easy to develop the habit of using food as a form of emotional fulfillment. It is also easy to believe that refusing food that is offered when you are not hungry or which you prefer not to eat might be interpreted as refusing the love that motivated the offer.

Like so many people, I have been dealing with food addictions for most of my life. In my family, I learned very early to equate food with love. While on the one hand food was treated as an expression of love and family togetherness, on the other hand my mother often encouraged me to lose weight. When I was a schoolgirl, my lunch bag would be full of celery, carrot sticks, and cottage cheese, while all my friends would have nice–looking sandwiches and cookies for dessert. I developed the habit of sneaking out to buy hamburgers, French fries, and milkshakes to express my rebellion.

As I began my quest for better health, I knew I had to get rid of my obsessive feelings about food. Realizing that I was using food as physical nourishment, I begin to look for other things that were nurturing for me. Getting a massage, talking with a close friend, going to the movies, or walking by the ocean are some of the things that now provide the emotional support I used to seek in food. I look for uplifting options when I am upset or burned out or bored, and instead of turning to food, I can choose one of these other outlets to gratify myself.

During the 21–Day Program, you will discover that relaxing baths, besides all their other health benefits, are a wonderful source of emotional support. For example, the Tranquility Bath on page 156 will provide an opportunity for you to lie back and reflect on what kinds of things nurture you. At the same time, the Cucumber Cleansing Facial and the Yogurt Toning Mask will show you that many foods can be beneficial outside the body as well as inside.

Think about the things that nurture you. If you wish, write them in your journal. List the things that you know give you physical and emotional comfort–perhaps puttering in your garden, listening to music, or curling up with a pot of peppermint tea and a good book. As you go through the Cleansing and Rejuvenation Program, you will probably discover some new activities that you can add to your list. Keep this list up–to–date; it is a catalog of resources for those times that you might be tempted to turn to food for emotional gratification.

NOTES TO MYSELF

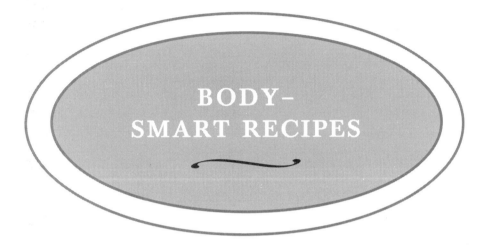

BODY–SMART RECIPES

*T*he following recipes are specially designed for use during the 21–Day Program. They contain no chemicals, preservatives, refined starches and sugars––no toxins of any kind. When you make these recipes, be sure to use organic produce or produce you have treated with the Cleansing Soak, and cold–pressed vegetable oils, to ensure that your meals are clean and clear.

Some of the ingredients may be unfamiliar to you. Part of the purpose of this program is to introduce you to the flavors and nutritional benefits of foods you may not have used before. I am sure that many will become life–long favorites.

DRINKS, TEAS, FLUSHES & OTHER MAGIC POTIONS

There is no better way to initiate the cleansing process than to begin to flush your body with the following beverages; they become an integral part of your Cleansing and Rejuvenation Program. Start out the morning with your first daily Hot Lemon–Water Flush, prepare a pot of Inner Beauty Herbal Tea to drink throughout the day, and you are on your way to cleaner, healthier cells and tissues. Be sure to use purified water for all the recipes I will be giving you. By eliminating the chemicals and other contaminants in tap water, you are already beginning to lighten the load of toxins in your body.

Hot Lemon–Water Flush

You will drink the Hot Lemon–Water Flush first thing each morning, to help complete the cleansing process that has been going on during the night. This drink flushes all the systems of elimination, especially the kidneys, the liver, and the colon. It helps to cleanse waste from the digestive tract and keep your breath sweet.

> 8–ounce glass of warm purified water
> Juice of 1/2 lemon
> Pinch of cayenne pepper

Heat eight ounces of purified water until it is quite warm, pour the water in a glass, and add the lemon juice and cayenne. You may increase the amount of cayenne gradually (up to one–eighth teaspoon) as you continue to make your Hot Lemon–Water Flush each morning. If the cayenne pepper is too stimulating for you in this form, you may use a 500 milligram cayenne capsule and take it with your Lemon–Water Flush.

Lemon juice helps to break up and dislodge the sticky mucus deposits that tend to clog up the system. Its powerful enzymes and high vitamin–C content are natural cleansers, helping to flush your system of toxic wastes. The bioflavonoid in the white inner rind and fibrous strands are also very cleansing, so use a squeezer to derive the benefits of these fibrous parts of the lemon as well. Cayenne pepper aids digestion by stimulating the production of digestive juices, and helps to eliminate mucus. It is healing to the respiratory system and is thought to enhance the effects of many other herbs and Vitamin C. Some people find that drinking hot water, even by itself, helps to encourage a bowel movement in the morning.

Inner Beauty Herbal Tea Blend

This blend was developed by Walt Baptiste of San Francisco. I have studied yoga and meditation with him for the last 20 years and have learned many wonderful practices from him, including this mineralizing tea.

You will enjoy the pleasantly soothing, minty taste of this tea as a daily beverage. Not only is it a delightful substitute for caffeine drinks, but it also promotes cleansing and nourishes the cells and tissues. Begin by making up a large batch of the dried herbs for the Herbal Tea Blend, so that you can use this pre–mixed blend each morning to prepare your tea.

> 1 cup dried peppermint
> 1/2 cup dried oat straw
> 1/2 cup dried alfalfa
> 1/2 cup dried sage

Combine all the herbs, mix together well, and store in an airtight container.

Each morning, boil four cups of purified water, remove it from the heat, and pour it into a teapot. Add four teaspoons of Herbal Tea Blend and steep for twenty minutes with the teapot covered. Strain the tea into a thermos or other container and drink it between meals throughout the day. You may reheat the tea if you wish, or drink it cold.

Peppermint is an excellent aid to digestion, and relieves flatulence and bowel spasms. Oat straw is rich in the mineral silica, an essential component of teeth, hair, skin, and nails. Oat straw tea is also a traditional remedy for chest ailments. Alfalfa is one of nature's richest sources of a variety of vitamins and minerals, including potassium and iron. Sage is an antispasmodic, and helps to eliminate mucus in the respiratory passages and stomach.

Hydrating Drink

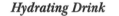

You can enhance the hydrating properties of your purified drinking water by adding a small amount of natural sugar. This Hydrating Drink was developed by two Australian doctors who were working in Africa with malnourished children. The doctors found that infants who were dehydrated from diarrhea were not helped when given water alone, but if some sugar was mixed in the water, it helped to rehydrate their tissues. Using sugar water for oral–hydration therapy is based on the same theory as giving intravenous glucose, or sugar water, to people in the hospital who cannot eat solid food.

You may prepare the Hydrating Drink using either pure maple syrup or apple juice, in the proportions given below. Be sure to use juice from organical-

FOCUS ON DAYS 2–21

ly grown apples, or pure maple syrup (not a maple–flavored, refined–sugar syrup). Both are excellent sweeteners. Try them, and see which suits your own taste.

6 ounces of purified water
2 ounces of organic apple juice

OR

8 ounces of purified water
1 teaspoon of pure maple syrup

Pour the pure maple syrup or apple juice into an empty glass and fill it to the top with purified water.

Drink a glass of Hydrating Drink between meals throughout the day, whenever you are thirsty. Bring some sweetener of your choice to work. Fill a glass with water from the cooler, add the sweetener, and sip it at your desk. This Hydrating Drink helps your body to absorb water at a cellular level. This keeps the tissues plump and moisturized, and promotes the cleansing activity of lymphatic fluid as water is moved in and out of the cells. Regular use of this Hydrating Drink keeps your system constantly flushed with fresh water, pushing the stagnant fluids out from between the cells and overcoming a tendency to bloating by removing salt. It also keeps your colon hydrated and discourages constipation.

If you are out and about during the day and do not have apple juice or maple syrup available, you may also use 2 ounces of Seven–Up in 6 ounces of purified water.

Oxygenation Cocktail

The Oxygenation Cocktail is a blend of minerals and powerful, space–age nutrients. This rich blend helps prepare your body for any kind of exercise by ensuring that all the muscles, tissues, and other cells are supplied with oxygen. The nutrients are absorbed very readily through the walls of the small intestine and colon. Drink this mixture just before you exercise each day.

To an eight ounce glass of purified water stir in:

> 1 Emergen–C packet or 1 teaspoon of vitamin–C powder
> 1 tablespoon liquid minerals
> Pinch of germanium (about 1/16 teaspoon)
> 1 ounce aloevera juice
> 1 tablespoon liquid chlorophyll

Along with this drink take:

> 10 drops of wheat–germ oil on the tongue
> 1 forty–milligram tablet of ginkgo–leaf extract
> 1 30 milligram capsule of co–enzyme Q–10

Emergen–C, which contains vitamin C and some minerals, can be purchased in any health–food store, or you can use powdered vitamin C (ascorbic acid). Vitamin C helps form collagen, so vital to repairing and rejuvenating the skin. Along with vitamin E and the trace mineral selenium, vitamin C is well known for its anti–aging action and preventing the accumulation of destructive free radicals in the cells.

Aloe vera juice, when taken internally, promotes cleansing of the digestive tract. It has also been reported helpful in the treatment of arthritis, allergies and strengthening the immune system. Externally, aloe vera juice is a remedy for burns, sunburn, skin irritation, and minor cuts and scratches. You may increase the amount of aloe vera in this recipe by one ounce per week, up to three ounces.

Liquid chlorophyll assists in the detoxification and healing of your digestive system.

Ginkgo–leaf extract is derived from an ancient species of tree native to China. Ginkgo–leaf has long been valued in Chinese herbal medicine and is just now being recognized in the West for its powerful anti–aging activity. Besides combating harmful free radicals, it helps to increase the flow of nutrients and oxygen to the circulatory system, eyes, ears, and brain.

Wheat–germ oil contains the active ingredient octacosanol. When taken just before you exercise, octacosanol exerts a powerful cleansing action, bringing oxygen into the muscle tissues and flushing the blood vessels.

Called the "nutrients of the nineties," co–enzyme Q–10 and germanium are being widely used in Japan. They are available in a number of forms–sublingual, powder, and capsules. All are equally effective.

Germanium has been nicknamed the "oxygen nutrient" because its oxygen–rich molecular structure facilitates the oxygenation of tissues. It also protects against harmful free radical molecules and stimulates the immune system. By increasing oxygenation, it promotes cell and tissue rejuvenation and improved metabolism. Due to FDA regulations, it is sometimes difficult to find Germanium. Watch for any changes in its availability.

Co–enzyme Q–10 protects against heart disease and high blood pressure, stimulates the immune system, slows the aging process, and guards against the gum disease that so often accompanies aging. As we grow older, our bodies become less capable of producing co–enzyme Q–10. Taking it as a supplement assists our cells and tissues in rejuvenating themselves. Co–enzyme Q–10 also helps athletes to meet their bodies' increased energy demands and can aid in weight loss because it increases the body's ability to burn stored fat.

You can benefit from these powerful health–promoting nutrients by adding them to your daily supplement program. The Oxygenation Cocktail, combined with exercise and correct breathing, will promote a dynamic oxygenating and cleansing action within your cells in a matter of minutes.

INNER BATHING: POLLUTION SOLUTIONS FOR INNER BEAUTY

At the same time that you are giving your system a rest by eating clean, simple foods, you will be using special beverages and herbal preparations to gently flush all of your systems of elimination and clean away the toxic debris. During your Cleansing and Rejuvenation Program, drinking large quantities of fluid, including generous quantities of your Hydrating Drink, is key. As you progress through the cleansing phase, you will add a powerful detoxifying herb, chaparral, to your Inner Beauty Herbal Tea Blend. On Day 10, the Inner Beauty Tea will be replaced by an Herbal Purification Tea that flushes the lymph system and removes congestion and toxicity from the digestive system. Also beginning on Day 10, you will start each morning with a Liver Flush, based on fruit juices, which helps trigger the liver to release stored toxins. To cleanse the kidneys and urinary system, you will drink a Diuretic Tea of special water–flushing herbs. All these beverages will be used during the cleansing period, along with an Intestinal Cleanser made up of fiber–rich seeds that will gently sweep and tone the intestinal tract.

For your convenience, many of these cleansing potions are already packaged and available at your local health–food store.

Inner Beauty Tea with Chaparral

---

2 tablespoons Inner Beauty Herbal Tea Blend (page 81)
2 teaspoons dried chaparral herb
6 cups purified water

Boil the water, remove from the heat, and add the Inner Beauty Tea Blend and the chaparral herb. Cover and steep for one hour, then strain it into a thermos or other container to drink, a cup at a time, throughout the day.

You may drink the tea cool, or you may warm it again if you wish. Sweeten the tea with a little honey if you want to.

Chaparral protects against infection and promotes elimination of toxins through the kidneys, lymph, and blood. It is a powerful herb used specifically for cleansing; it is not appropriate to drink as an everyday beverage.

Herbal Purification Tea

This pleasant tasting herbal flush helps to eliminate congestion and toxicity in the digestive and lymph systems.

1/4 cup of fennel seeds
1/4 cup of fenugreek seeks
1/4 cup of licorice root
1/2 cup of flax seeds
1/2 cup of peppermint leaves

Prepare a supply of Herbal Purification Tea blend by combining all ingredients and storing the mixture in an airtight container. To make a supply of the tea for the day, add four teaspoons of this blend to four cups of cold purified water, bring to a boil, and simmer, covered, for seven to ten minutes. Strain out the herbs and save the strained tea to drink at the specified times. You do not need to refrigerate the tea, and you may reheat it if you wish.

This tasty, fragrant herbal blend has powerful detoxifying effects, helping to expel mucus, remove gas from the intestines, promote digestion, cleanse the digestive system and the urinary tract, and soothe the mucous membranes. It is so effective at flushing the lymph system that people have reported a shrinking of swollen lymph nodes shortly after drinking this tea.

Liver Flush #1

This detoxifying drink which you will take several mornings during the cleansing phase helps to eliminate poisons stored in the liver. The liver filters pollutants out of the blood, but as long as more poisons are being put into the system, it does not have a chance to eliminate them all through the intestines. During a cleansing program, while you are giving your liver a rest, you can help flush the stored toxins out and restore its natural vitality.

juice of 1 to 2 lemons, freshly squeezed
juice of 1 orange, freshly squeezed
1 teaspoon of grated fresh ginger
pinch of cayenne pepper or 1 drop of cayenne tincture
1 to 3 cloves garlic, crushed
1 tablespoon safflower oil, cold–pressed
1 tablespoon olive oil, cold–pressed

Combine all the ingredients and drink the Liver Flush early in the morning. Do not eat anything for two hours, to allow this potent flush to act undisturbed by food in your body. During this two–hour period, drink Herbal Purification Tea to support the cleansing process.

Begin with a pinch of cayenne pepper or a drop of cayenne tincture, and increase gradually as you get used to the hot taste, up to no more than one–eighth teaspoon of the powder or eight drops of the tincture. Do not use more of the cayenne than is pleasant and comfortable for you. You may also begin with a smaller amount of ginger and gradually increase it to one teaspoon or more, and with one clove of garlic, increasing to three.

Liver Flush #1 amplifies the benefits of the Hot Lemon–Water Flush you begin drinking in the first week of the Program. The addition of orange juice enriches the drink with an extra boost of vitamin C, a powerful protective cleanser. The white inner peel and fibrous strands of the orange contain cleansing bioflavonoids, so be sure to include some in the juice. Do not worry if you get some seeds in the juice; they contain beneficial enzymes, vitamins, and minerals, and stimulate the liver and gallbladder. Orange juice helps combat viruses, lowers blood cholesterol, and reduces the risk of some kinds of cancer. Garlic promotes the detoxifying activity of the liver, and olive oil stimulates the secretion of bile, flushing out the liver though the hepatic duct.

Liver Flush #2

On varying mornings, you will drink another liver–flushing beverage, based on organic apples. Apple juice contains malic acid, which helps to cleanse the intestines and heal inflammation of the mucous membranes. If you do not have a juicer, look for fresh organic apple juice in the refrigerator section of your health–food store. Do not use commercial juice or nonorganic apples, since they may add to the toxic load on your liver.

> 1 cup of organic apple juice, freshly made
> juice of two lemons, freshly squeezed
> 1 teaspoon of grated fresh ginger
> pinch of cayenne pepper or 1 drop of cayenne tincture
> 1 to 3 cloves garlic, crushed
> 1 tablespoon of safflower oil, cold–pressed
> 1 tablespoon of olive oil, cold–pressed

Combine all the ingredients and drink early in the morning. Do not eat anything for two hours, to allow the Liver Flush to stimulate the detoxification of the liver. During this two–hour period, drink Herbal Purification Tea to support the cleansing process.

You may increase the amount of cayenne pepper, ginger, and garlic, as described in Liver Flush #1.

Diuretic Tea

The combination of special herbs in the Diuretic Tea promotes cleansing through the kidneys and bladder. It helps to relieve the water retention that often lies at the root of premenstrual stress, and will overcome uncomfortable and unsightly bloating. Juniper berries and uva–ursi leaves are well known for their diuretic effects. Parsley root is a remedy for water retention as well as for ailments of the liver and gallbladder. Licorice root imparts a sweet taste to the tea and soothes the mucous membranes of the urinary passages. During Week 2, you will drink one cup of Diuretic Tea one hour before dinner.

---

3 tablespoons of juniper berries, crushed
3 tablespoons of uva–ursi leaves
3 tablespoons of licorice root
3 tablespoons of parsley root

Prepare a supply of this Diuretic Tea blend by combining all ingredients and storing in an airtight container. To make a cup of tea, add one teaspoon of this blend to one cup of boiling water, cover, and let it steep for fifteen to thirty minutes. Strain out the herbs and drink the strained tea.

Intestinal Cleanser

Seeds and their hulls are an excellent source of the fiber that helps to cleanse the bowels. On contact with water, the mucilaginous seed coatings swell, softening the stool and helping it to move quickly and easily through the colon. Every day during Week 2, you will be taking an intestinal cleanser before bedtime, so that it can gently sweep out your digestive tract while you sleep.

If you have the time, I suggest that you make your own intestinal cleanser to use in the 21–Day Program. The seeds and husks, ground to a powder, are available in bulk in health–food stores.

1/2 teaspoon psyllium husks, powdered
1 teaspoon flax seed, powdered
4 to 6 ounces of purified water

Add the psyllium husks and flax seed to the water and stir thoroughly. The consistency of the mixture will change as it begins to gel. Use enough water so that you can swallow the mixture easily. Drink it all at one time; you will notice that the flax seeds impart a slightly nutlike flavor.

If you prefer, you may purchase an intestinal cleanser at a health–food store. There are many good brands of ready–mixed intestinal cleansers on the market. These products generally contain a combination of seeds, including psyllium and flax, and sometimes beneficial bacteria as well. If you use a commercially prepared product, be sure to follow the instructions on the package.

Apple-Cider Vinegar Drink

Apple–cider vinegar is a popular folk remedy for aiding the digestion process. It is believed to be a supplement for the hydrochloric acid in the stomach, helping the digestion of proteins and the absorption of minerals and vitamins B and C.

1 teaspoon apple–cider vinegar
1/2 teaspoon honey with royal jelly
2 ounces purified water

Combine all ingredients and drink before eating a protein meal. You can make up a mixture of the vinegar and honey and take it with you to work. Add purified water to the basic mixture and drink a glass before you go to lunch.

Rejuvelac

Rejuvelac is a fermented grain drink. It has been valued by women for centuries for its ability to impart a beautiful complexion. Furthermore, Rejuvelac is high in the friendly bacteria that are so important for a healthy colon. The tonic can be made from either wheatberries, rye, barley or millet. The taste varies depending on which grain is used. Barley is my personal favorite; it imparts a nutlike flavor to the Rejuvelac and is delightfully fragrant as it ferments. Millet has a tangy, lemony flavor. Experiment to find a taste that you enjoy.

1 cup of wheatberries, rye, barley or millet
1 quart of purified water

Soak the raw grain in water for twenty–four hours without refrigerating. After twenty–four hours, pour off the water and refrigerate it to drink throughout the day as a refreshing and rejuvenating between–meal beverage. If any beverage is left over at the end of the day, add it to your bath water, and prepare a new batch of Rejuvelac for tomorrow. Reuse the grain base at least three times, and up to five times, if you wish.

CLEANSING SOAK FOR FRUITS AND VEGETABLES

You may not be able to purchase organically grown produce. Don't worry, you can remove harmful contaminants from your fruits and vegetables by using the following cleansing soak. This soak not only purifies your produce, but it also helps it to stay fresh longer.

Travelers and American families stationed abroad have traditionally used a Clorox soak to cleanse fruits and vegetables of sprays, bacteria, viruses, parasites, and toxic metals. The active ingredient in this bleach product causes allergic reactions in many people. That is why I recommend a more recent idea: the hydrogen–peroxide soak. Hydrogen peroxide is a common antiseptic that many people use as an external germ-killer. Dentists recommend hydrogen peroxide solution for cleansing teeth and controlling gum disease.

If you have a water purifier, use purified water for this soak; if not, you may use tap water.

1/4 cup of 3 percent hydrogen peroxide (drugstore variety)
2 gallons of water (about a dishpan full)

Fill a dishpan or other container with the water and add the hydrogen peroxide. Soak thin–skinned fruits (berries, peaches, apricots) or leafy vegetables in this cleansing bath for fifteen minutes. Soak thick–skinned fruits (apples, citrus) or fibrous, thick–skinned, or root vegetables for thirty minutes. It is okay to combine fruits and vegetables of the same type.

Remove the fruits and vegetables from the cleansing bath and let them stand in clear purified water for ten minutes. Then drain them, dry them thoroughly, and store in the usual manner.

BODY-SMART BREAKFASTS

Fresh Apple Breakfast

This old adage about "an apple a day" has a basis in fact. Researchers have found that people who added two or three apples a day to their diet showed a 10 percent decrease in their blood–cholesterol levels. Apples contain a fruit fiber known as pectin, which helps to sweep out and detoxify the alimentary canal. Pectin is the active ingredient in the pharmaceutical Kaopectate, a classic over–the–counter remedy for diarrhea.

Apples provide sweetness while keeping blood sugar on an even keel, and aid in controlling appetite by producing a satisfying feeling of fullness. They are also good for cleansing the teeth and stimulating the gums.

If you possibly can, buy organic apples that are free of pesticides and other chemicals. Apples grown with chemicals have toxins even in the core! Many supermarkets are now beginning to carry apples and other produce that have not been sprayed. Choose your favorite sweet red apples (I prefer Red Delicious), and eat them raw, up to three small apples or two large ones. Be sure to eat the skin, which is very high in pectin fiber. Some people even like to eat the seeds, because of their rich supply of nutrients.

Healing Grape Breakfast

Grapes have long enjoyed a popular reputation as a healing fruit. In the late 1920's, grapes were in vogue when a South African woman, Johanna Brandt, wrote a book claiming that she had cured her abdominal cancer with a grape diet and grape packs. The high levels of caffeic acid in grapes may explain their reported anticancer action, although no studies have been done using humans. Grapes, grape juice, raisins, and grape–based wines have been shown to kill disease–causing viruses in test–tube experiments. Best of all, grapes taste wonderful. Eat as many as you wish for a breakfast rich in natural sugars and cleansing enzymes. Be sure to choose organically raised grapes, or cleanse them thoroughly with the Cleansing Soak for Fruits and Vegetables to remove contaminating sprays.

Fresh Pineapple Breakfast

Choose a fresh pineapple that is very, very ripe, so that it doesn't irritate the mouth. Slice and eat as much as you want. Fresh pineapple contains the enzyme bromelain, which interacts with stomach acid to digest excess protein and burn body fat.

Many digestive upset problems can be alleviated by providing the body with enzymes to help break down undigested proteins and other food residues. I recommend the use of a digestive–enzyme supplement whenever you mis-combine foods or eat too much protein. The bromelain in pineapple works much the same as the enzymes in the human digestive system. For this reason, pineapple is a great cleansing meal for any day after you have indulged in too much rich food. Fresh pineapple juice is also a helpful home remedy for reliving sore, raspy throats.

Papaya Complexion Breakfast

Papaya is a delicious tropical fruit with an incomparable flavor and unsurpassed nutritional value. Richer in nutrients than just about any other fruit, papaya has an abundance of vitamins A, C, D, E, and K, as well as the minerals calcium, phosphorus, and iron. Papaya contains hardly any starch; it is made up of simple, natural sugars that are readily absorbed into the bloodstream. Not only has nature already broken down its sugars, but the papaya enzyme papain also helps in the digestion of other foods. This is such a powerful enzyme that the American Indians wrapped meat in the leaves of the papaya plant in order to tenderize it.

Papaya is very good food for digestive disorders, because it can be tolerated by the stomach when other foods cannot. It cuts excessive mucoid material that accumulates in the digestive tract, aids in breaking down proteins and other hard–to–digest foods, helps to cleanse the intestinal tract of decayed matter, and promotes regular elimination. It even protects against bad breath and offensive body odors, and cleans the mouth and teeth.

Select a large ripe papaya, cut it in half, and scoop out the seeds. Then you may either scoop out the flesh with a spoon, or peel it and eat it in slices. Eat as much as you want, up to one whole papaya.

Berry Breakfast

The high fiber content of berries sweeps the intestinal walls of toxic wastes. Their rich mineral content has earned them a reputation as potent blood purifiers. When you add their sweet–tart flavor to their health benefits, you have an irresistible concoction.

> 1/2 pint strawberries, sliced or halved
> 1/4 cup fresh orange juice
> 1/2 cup blueberries or raspberries

Soak the sliced strawberries in orange juice for fifteen to thirty minutes. Puree the blueberries or raspberries in a blender or food processor and pour the topping over the strawberries.

Strawberries are valued for their blood–cleansing properties owing to their high vitamin–C and mineral content. They have been used for disorders of the intestinal tract, liver, heart, and kidneys, and for gout and rheumatic problems. They have also been used as a dentifrice. High in the fruit fiber pectin, strawberries help to lower blood cholesterol. Recent research indicates that people who eat strawberries have a reduced incidence of cancer. Strawberries have also been found to help kill disease–causing viruses.

Blueberries kill both viruses and bacteria, owing to compounds called anthocyanosides, which may also protect against heart disease and stroke by preventing cholesterol from penetrating blood–vessel walls, especially in the brain. Blueberries are a popular folk remedy for diarrhea.

Raspberries are a mild intestinal cleanser. Raspberry–leaf tea is a great traditional "female remedy" used to relieve nausea in pregnancy, ease childbirth, and reduce menstrual cramps.

Fresh Cantaloupe Breakfast

Cantaloupe has been valued by people all over the world as a healing fruit. In China, it is used to treat hepatitis; in the Philippines, to treat cancer and induce menstruation; in India, as a diuretic; and in Guatemala, the seeds are used to expel worms. Such traditional uses of cantaloupe are now being authenticated by scientific research. Like other orange–colored fruits, cantaloupe is high in beta–carotene and other carotenoids, which are believed to aid in the prevention of cancer, according to epidemiological studies comparing diets and cancer rates.

Recent medical findings show that cantaloupe also helps to inhibit blood clotting, thereby protecting against heart disease and stroke. The chemical believed responsible for this anticlotting effect is adenosine, the same compound that accounts, at least in part, for the similar anticoagulant action of garlic and onions.

Like all melons, cantaloupe is very high in water content. Because it moves out of the stomach very quickly, it should not be eaten in combination with other fruits. Eat one–half to one whole fresh cantaloupe for breakfast. The high water soluble–fiber content are extremely effective for cleansing the digestive tract.

> ### *Cleansing Watermelon Breakfast*

Watermelon is filled with sweet water, and when eaten alone for breakfast it helps to flush the entire digestive system. It is the breakfast of choice at some of the cleansing–oriented spas. Eat as much watermelon as you wish. This fun fruit breakfast completes your body's natural nocturnal cleansing process.

SOUPS AND BROTHS

> ### *Potassium Broth*

Potassium Broth is one of the mainstays of your 21–Day Program. It is delicious all by itself, either thin or thick, hot or cold. You will also be using it as a stock for nourishing vegetable soups. It is rich in minerals and is the quintessential cleanser for the intestines and the blood.

You will use my Potassium Broth recipe to make both a thick bisque for a satisfying meal, and strained to make a thin broth. The thin broth will be used as a base for other soups, and as a mineral–rich drink during the cleansing phase of the program.

14 carrots, with tops
14 celery stalks, with tops
Beet tops from 2 bunches
4 potatoes
2 onions

4 cloves of garlic
3 summer squash
3 zucchini
2 handfuls of parsley

1. Chop all of the vegetables, place them in an eight–quart soup pot.

2. Cover the vegetables with purified water.

3. Bring the water to a boil and turn the heat down to a simmer.

4. Simmer uncovered, for thirty minutes.

5. Turn off the heat and allow the broth to sit, covered, for another thirty minutes.

6. Remove the greens from the pot and discard them. The nutrients from the greens are now in the stock.

7. Remove the rest of the vegetables from the broth and put them into a food processor or blender to puree them. (Depending on the size of your appliance, you may need to do this in batches.) Add one–fourth cup of the liquid broth to each pureed batch. You may keep adding broth, a bit at a time, until the puree is the consistency you like.

8. Empty each batch from your blender or processor into a storage container for your refrigerator.

9. Put the rest of the clear broth into a separate container to use as a base for your other soups or as a quick pick–me–up between meals.

Helpful Hints

* Both the thick bisque and the thin broth can be stored in the refrigerator for up to five days. You may wish to make a double batch of the recipe and freeze it in four–cup containers to be used throughout the program. (If you do this, you will need to use a larger pot.)

* Take either the bisque or broth along with you in your thermos to use as a midafternoon snack, or have a cup of the nourishing mixture before going to bed.

Variations

* Add a packet of Knox unflavored gelatin to a cup of the broth or bisque to add protein richness. The gelatin will also assist the absorption of vitamins and minerals into your system.

* Add one tablespoon of granulated lecithin to each cup of bisque or broth for additional cleansing power.

* Add additional cloves of garlic to your soup pot as desired.

* If desired, add one bunch of spinach as well.

* For a different flavor and extra nutrition, dissolve one–half to one teaspoon of miso in one–fourth cup of hot broth and add it to your bowl of bisque or cup of broth.

MINERALIZING SOUPS

The following vegetable–soup recipes use Potassium Broth as a base. Take any of these delicious bisques along with you in a thermos for a quick, satisfying lunch or snack on a busy day; or combine them with a salad for a complete evening meal. These recipes provide four small or two large servings. The yield for each recipe is given in terms of small servings, the equivalent of side dishes. If you are going to use the dish as a main course, the yield is half as many servings. These recipes are free of fattening and hard–to–digest ingredients, so do not hesitate to eat as large a helping as you wish. You can also freeze separate portions for later on in the program.

Squash Bisque
(Serves 4)

---

1 medium butternut squash or acorn squash
1 onion
1 tablespoon olive oil
2 tablespoons sweet white miso
4 cups Potassium Broth
2 tablespoons granulated lecithin
1/4 teaspoon ginger or curry (to taste)

1. Cube the squash and place it in a pot with the Potassium Broth.

2. Bring it to a quick boil and turn it down immediately.

3. Simmer for 15 to 20 minutes.

4. While the squash is simmering, slice the onion and saute it in the olive oil until it is golden.

5. Add the onion to the squash.

6. Add ginger or curry, your choice.

7. Continue simmering for another 10 minutes or until the squash is soft.

8. Let it sit for another 15 minutes.

9. Remove 1/4 cup of broth and dissolve the miso in it. Set aside for a moment.

10. Transfer the soup into a food processor or blender and puree. Add the lecithin and miso broth just as you are finishing.

11. Garnish with a handful of chopped parsley, toasted almond slivers, toasted sesame seeds, chopped scallions, or nori flakes.

Helpful Hints

* Winter squashes like butternut squash are fairly starchy and should not be combined with protein. They may be combined with salad or cooked vegetables for a complete Clean and Clear meal.

Carrot Bisque
(Serves 4)

8 carrots
2 potatoes
1 onion
1/4 teaspoon grated ginger
4 cups Potassium Broth
2 tablespoons granulated lecithin

Follow cooking and preparation instructions for Squash Bisque.

Cauliflower Bisque
(Serves 4)

1 head cauliflower
2 potatoes
1 yellow onion
1 clove garlic, minced
1/4 teaspoon curry
4 cups Potassium Broth
2 tablespoons granulated lecithin

Follow cooking and preparation instructions for Squash Bisque.

Yam Delight
(Serves 4)

2 yams
1 large onion
1 tablespoon olive oil
2 cloves garlic, minced
1 tablespoon fresh grated ginger
2 cups Potassium Broth or purified water
1 handful parsley, chopped
sea salt to taste

1.   Bake the yams at 350 degrees until they are soft.

2.   While the yams are baking, chop the onion and saute it in the olive oil with the garlic and ginger until the onion is translucent.

3.   Peel and cube the baked yams.

4. Place the yams and the sauteed onion mixture in a blender or food processor.

5. Puree the mixture while slowly adding the Potassium Broth.

6. Garnish with chopped parsley and add sea salt to taste.

Helpful Hints

* Yams are a starchy food, and should not be combined with protein. Combine this bisque with a salad or steamed vegetables.

Variations

* Yam Delight is a delicious topping for steamed vegetables; reduce the amount of Potassium Broth to create a thick mixture.

Beet Borscht
(Serves 4)

---

1 bunch fresh beets
2 carrots
1 onion
1 teaspoon caraway seeds
1 tablespoon olive oil
2 cups Potassium Broth
1 cup nonfat yogurt
juice of 1/2 lemon
pinch of sea salt

1. Trim the greens from the beets and save them for your next batch of Potassium Broth. Scrub the beets well.

2. Place the beets in 2 inches of water in a covered pot. Bake them at 350 degrees for about an hour, until soft. Check occasionally to be sure the water has not evaporated, and add a bit more water if necessary.

3. While the beets are cooling, slice the carrots and onions.

4. Saute them in olive oil with the caraway seeds at a very low temperature until the carrots are soft and the onions are golden.

5. Drain and cool the beets.

6. Slip off the skins with your fingers and slice the beets.

7. Place all of the ingredients except lemon juice and salt into a blender or food processor. Puree while slowly adding the Potassium Broth and yogurt.

8. Add the lemon juice and sea salt to taste.

9. Return the borscht to a pan, heat it slowly, and serve.

Helpful Hints

* Because this soup contains yogurt, it is a protein dish and should not be combined with starches.

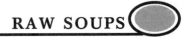

Variations

* Serve Beet Borscht chilled if desired.

* During the cleansing phase of the program, you may delete the yogurt and add an additional cup of Potassium Broth.

RAW SOUPS

These delicious uncooked vegetable soups will be featured during Week 2. These soups are a potent source for all the vitamins and minerals available in the raw vegetables themselves. Their fiber content helps to sweep the intestines of waste, assisting the intense cleansing that takes place during the second week of the program.

Raw Vegetable Delight
(Serves 4)

---

2 1/2 cups tomatoes, chopped
2 cloves garlic, minced
4 cups onion, chopped
2 cucumbers, peeled and sliced
2 yellow squash, chopped
2 zucchini, chopped
2 cups celery, diced
4 cups red bell pepper, diced
1 ear of corn
4 teaspoons sea salt
1 tablespoon umeboshi vinegar
1 tablespoon dried dill or 2 tablespoons fresh dill

1. Cut the corn off the cob and combine it with all the other ingredients in a blender or food processor.

2. Puree the mixture and pour it into a serving bowl.

3. Garnish the soup with thin slices of cucumber and a sprinkle of fresh dill.

Raw Vegetable "Cream" Soup
(Serves 4)

---

1 1/2 cups carrots, chopped
2 cloves garlic, minced
1 cup alfalfa sprouts

1 tablespoon olive oil
1 tablespoon Herbamare
2 cups Potassium Broth
1 avocado, diced
pinch of nori flakes, as garnish

1. Blend the first six ingredients in a blender or food processor.
2. Add the avocado and blend again for a few seconds.
3. Pour the mixture into a serving bowl and garnish it with nori flakes.

Helpful Hints

* These raw soups are excellent for tasty hot–weather meals after you have completed the 21–Day Program.

Variations

* Substitute broccoli, cauliflower, or spinach for the carrots for a different taste treat.

* Combine carrots, broccoli, cauliflower, and spinach together for a mixed vegetable soup that is packed with nutrients.

MIRACLE SALADS

These salads are excellent sources of vitamins and minerals. Adding a salad dressing containing GLA–rich oils helps to ensure healthy skin, hair, and nails and to control cholesterol levels in your blood.

To provide a daily helping of miracle foods and anti–aging vegetables, you will eat the Super Salad regularly during the 21–Day Program. Later on, make it a part of your lifetime eating habits. Combine these salads with either a protein or a starchy food for a complete meal. These recipes provide four small or two large servings. The yield for each recipe is given in terms of small servings, the equivalent of side dishes. If you are going to use the dish as a main course, the yield is half as many servings. These recipes are free of fattening and hard–to–digest ingredients, so do not hesitate to eat as large a helping as you wish.

> *Super Salad*
> *(Serves 4)*

2 cups mixed sprouts (sprouted sunflower seeds,
mung beans, alfalfa seeds, garbanzo beans, lentils,

radishes, and wheat berries.)
8 cups organic mixed greens (do not include
iceberg lettuce. It is difficult to digest and tends to
be constipating)
1/2 red and/or green cabbage, shredded
2 carrots, grated
1 zucchini, grated
1/2 pound broccoli, broken into flowerets
1 sliced cucumber
garlic, minced, up to 2 cloves
granulated lecithin, 2 tablespoons
1/2 cup sunflower and pumpkin seeds, hulled and
unsalted (optional, as a protein source)

1. Steam the broccoli and the cauliflower.

2. Toss the first seven ingredients together in a large salad bowl.

3. When ready to serve, top with the sliced cucumber, minced garlic, lecithin, and seeds.

4. Toss the salad with the Fat–Loss Dressing of your choice (pages 100 to 101) and serve immediately.

Helpful Hints

* This recipe provides 4 generous servings. You may make up enough for 2–3 days and store it in an airtight container in the refrigerator.

* Many health–food stores and quality supermarkets now carry prewashed, mixed salad greens. They also have many of the sprouts. This makes it much easier to prepare your salad.

* Do not add the garlic, cucumber, lecithin, sunflower or pumpkin seeds, or salad dressing until you are ready to serve the salad.

* Vary the garlic to suit your taste. Try to build up to 2 minced cloves per serving. If you prefer, you may get your garlic from the salad dressing. Remember, you may chew fresh parsley after eating garlic to mask the odor.

* If you are having the Super Salad as a complete meal or combining it with a steamed vegetable dish, add the sunflower seeds and/or pumpkin seeds to provide excellent protein. Omit the seeds if you are combining the salad with a protein or starchy dish such as Yam Delight.

High–Iron Salad
(Serves 4)

---

1 bunch beets
1 bunch watercress
Lemon–Mustard Dressing (page 101)

1. Trim the greens from the beets and save them for your next batch of

Potassium Broth. Scrub the beets well.

2.   Place the beets in 2 inches of water in a covered pot. Bake them at 350 degrees for about an hour, until soft. Check occasionally to be sure the water has not evaporated, and add a bit more water if necessary.

3.   Drain and cool the beets.

4.   Slip off the skins with your fingers and slice the beets.

5.   Wash the watercress well, remove large stems and wilted leaves, and arrange it on a plate.

6.   Place the beets over the bed of watercress.

7.   Top with Lemon–Mustard Dressing.

FAT-LOSS DRESSINGS

These salad and vegetable dressings help to flush fat from your system because of the beneficial omega–6, or GLA, oils in safflower and sesame oil. Be sure to use cold–pressed vegetable oils to ensure that you are deriving the full benefits of the GLA oils. Make up a batch of your favorite Fat–Loss Dressing and store it in your refrigerator. Take some with you in a small container when you go to a restaurant, and you will always be able to enjoy a healthy, properly combined salad. (If you forget, you can request olive oil and lemon or vinegar on the side.)

Helpful Hints

* To make a creamier dressing or a tangy dip, add 1/4 to 1/2 cup of yogurt or 2 to 4 ounces of tofu to any of these recipes. Remember that the dressing is then a protein food; do not combine it with other proteins or with starches.

Garlic–Tarragon Dressing
(Serves 4)

> 1/3 cup safflower oil
> 3 garlic cloves, minced
> 1/2 teaspoon tarragon
> 2 tablespoons balsamic vinegar
> pinch of sea salt

Place all ingredients in a blender and blend thoroughly. Store the extra dressing in a glass jar in the refrigerator.

Raspberry–Vinaigrette Dressing
(Serves 4)

3 tablespoons olive oil
2 tablespoons safflower oil
1 tablespoon raspberry vinegar
1 teaspoon umeboshi vinegar
juice of 1 lemon
Herbamare to taste
1 clove garlic, minced
1/8 cup fresh parsley, chopped
pinch of peppermint
dash of pepper

Place all ingredients in a blender and blend thoroughly. Store the extra dressing in a glass jar in the refrigerator.

Lemon–Mustard Dressing
(Serves 4)

juice of 1/2 lemon
2 tablespoons tahini
1 tablespoon olive oil
1 tablespoon safflower oil
1/2 tablespoon brown–rice miso
1 teaspoon Dijon mustard
1/8 cup Potassium Broth
1 teaspoon honey

Place all ingredients in a blender and blend thoroughly. Store the extra dressing in a glass jar in the refrigerator.

Variations

* Lemon–Mustard Dressing is delicious heated and poured over steamed vegetables.

Lemon–Parsley Dressing
(Serves 4)

1/4 cup sesame oil
1/4 cup safflower oil
2 tablespoons brown–rice vinegar

1/2 cup chopped parsley
juice of 1/2 lemon
1 teaspoon sweet white miso
handful of toasted sunflower seeds

Place all ingredients in a blender and blend thoroughly. Store the extra dressing in a glass jar in the refrigerator.

CLEAN AND CLEAR TOPPINGS

These Clean and Clear toppings are divided into two groups. The first five are based on vegetables, and may be combined with starches and proteins as well as with vegetables. The last four are made with protein. These should be used as toppings for vegetables, but should not be combined with other proteins or with starches. These recipes provide four small or two large servings. The yield for each recipe is given in terms of small servings, the equivalent of side dishes. If you are going to use the dish as a main course, the yield is half as many servings. These recipes are free of fattening and hard–to–digest ingredients, so do not hesitate to eat as large a helping as you wish.

Helpful Hints

* All the Clean and Clear Toppings may be kept in the refrigerator for up to three days.

> *Green Goddess Topping*
> *(Serves 4)*

1 cup broccoli, divided into flowerets and steamed
1/8 cup olive oil
1/8 cup fresh basil
1 clove garlic, minced
1 teaspoon sweet white miso
Herbamare to taste

1. Steam the broccoli.
2. Combine all ingredients in a blender and blend until creamy.

Golden Goddess Topping
(Serves 4)

1 small butternut squash
1 carrot
1 clove garlic
1/2 tablespoon brown rice miso

1. Cut the squash into large pieces.

2. Place the cut–up squash in a pot with the carrot and garlic and cover with purified water.

3. Boil until the squash is tender (about 20 minutes).

4. Drain and reserve the water.

5. Scoop the flesh of the squash out of the skin.

6. Place the vegetables in a blender and puree. Add a little of the cooking water if necessary to create a smooth consistency.

Spa Salsa
(Serves 4)

3 tablespoons cilantro
1/4 cup green bell pepper, chopped
1/4 cup red bell pepper, chopped
1 tomato, chopped
1/2 red onion, chopped
2 scallions, chopped
juice of 1 lemon
1 garlic clove, minced

Combine all the ingredients in a bowl and toss. This recipe makes a delicious topping for fish as well as for steamed and raw vegetables.

Variations

* Add 1 diced jalapeno pepper to make a spicy salsa topping.

Carrot–Leek Puree
(Serves 4)

3 cups sliced carrots
1 cup sliced leeks
dill to taste

fresh lemon juice to taste
sea salt to taste

1. Steam the carrots until just tender (10 to 15 minutes, depending on the maturity of the carrots).

2. Add the leeks to the carrots and steam until the leeks have wilted.

3. Transfer the vegetables to a blender or food processor and puree until smooth.

4. Season the puree with a pinch of dill, sea salt, and a few drops of fresh lemon juice to taste.

Variations

* Substitute steamed white turnips for the carrots to make a sweet, high–potassium and high–calcium topping.

* Use carrots and turnips together for another variation.

Warm Garlic Dressing
(Serves 4)

---

2 tablespoons olive oil
2 tablespoons sliced garlic
3 tablespoons red–wine vinegar or lemon juice

1. Warm all ingredients in a small saucepan for 5 minutes.

2. Pour the dressing immediately over freshly steamed vegetables, or pour it over raw spinach or lettuce to create a "wilted" salad.

Helpful Hints

* This quick and easy dressing is a great way to add a healthy dose of garlic topping to your cooked vegetables.

Tahini–Tofu Topping
(Serves 4)

---

4 ounces tofu
2 tablespoons tahini
1 tablespoon brown–rice vinegar
1/8 cup Potassium Broth or purified water
2 scallions, chopped
1 tablespoon sesame oil
1 tablespoon umeboshi vinegar
pinch of sea salt

Combine all ingredients in a blender and blend until smooth.

Helpful Hints

* The tahini in this recipe imparts a nut–like sesame taste and provides beneficial GLA oils.

Carrot–Yogurt Topping
(Serves 4)

1 cup yogurt
1 tablespoon honey
1 tablespoon grated onion
1 tablespoon apple cider vinegar
1 carrot, grated

Combine all ingredients in a blender and blend until smooth.

Tofu–Ginger Topping
(Serves 4)

8 ounces tofu
2 tablespoons sesame oil
2–1/2 tablespoons brown–rice vinegar
1 tablespoon toasted sesame oil
1–1/2 tablespoons sweet white miso
1 tablespoon sesame seeds
1 tablespoon chopped fresh parsley
pinch of sea salt
1/2 teaspoon fresh grated ginger, garnish

Combine all the ingredients except the ginger in a blender and blend until smooth. Spoon the topping over raw or cooked vegetables and garnish with the fresh grated ginger.

Tofu–Miso Topping
(Serves 4)

1/4 cup Potassium Broth
8 ounces tofu
1 to 1–1/2 tablespoons brown–rice miso
1 tablespoon sesame oil

Combine all ingredients in a blender and blend until smooth.

Helpful Hints

* This is my favorite dip for raw and steamed vegetables.

SEA–VEGETABLE SPECIALTIES

These sea–vegetable recipes are rich in iodine, a nutrient essential to proper functioning of the thyroid gland and the regulation of the metabolism. Seaweed also contains a wealth of other trace minerals found in the ocean. You will use these recipes during Week 3 of the program. The hijiki and wakame called for in these recipes are dried seaweeds. They can be purchased in a health–food store, a Japanese food store, or in the Oriental foods section of a well–stocked supermarket. These recipes provide four small or two large servings. The yield for each recipe is given in terms of small servings, the equivalent of side dishes. If you are going to use the dish as a main course, the yield is half as many servings.

Hijiki Stir–Fry
(Serves 4)

1/2 cup hijiki
1 tablespoon sesame oil
2 cloves garlic, minced
1 tablespoon grated ginger
1/2 onion, chopped
1/2 cup celery, chopped
1 cup carrots, chopped
1 cup broccoli, broken into flowerets, and/or
chopped cabbage
juice of 1/2 lemon
1 tablespoon tamari
1/4 cup purified water
1 teaspoon maple syrup
1 tablespoon mirin (sweet cooking sake)
1 tablespoon white sesame seeds, to garnish

1. Rinse and soak the hijiki for 15 minutes.

2. Heat the sesame oil in a frying pan or wok.

3. Add the garlic, ginger, and onion. Saute until the onions are translucent (about 2 minutes).

4. Add the hijiki, celery, carrots, broccoli and/or cabbage, and continue to saute.

---

5.   Mix the lemon juice, tamari, water, maple syrup, and mirin, and add them to the vegetables.

6.   Simmer, covered, for 5 minutes.

7.   Spoon the stir–fry into a serving dish. Garnish it with raw sesame seeds and serve it immediately.

Variation

* Allow the Hijiki Stir–Fry to cool and spoon it over a bed of organic greens and shredded cabbage for a tasty, iodine–rich salad.

Miso Sea Soup
(Serves 4)

4 cups Potassium Broth
2 or 3 dried shitake mushrooms
1/2 cup wakame
8 ounces tofu
3 tablespoons brown–rice miso
2 scallions, chopped

1.   Soak the mushrooms in 1 cup of purified water for 10 minutes. Cut off and discard the stems and slice the mushrooms into thin strips.

2.   Soak the wakame in enough water to cover for 10 minutes.

3.   Bring the Potassium Broth to a boil in a 3–quart soup pot.

4.   Reduce the heat to a simmer and add the mushrooms and wakame. Cook, covered, for 7 minutes.

5.   While the soup is cooking, cut the tofu into cubes. Add it to the soup and cook, covered, for another 5 minutes.

6.   Thin the miso with a few tablespoons of the cooking broth and add it to the soup, stirring it until smooth.

7.   Remove the soup from the heat immediately.

8.   Serve and garnish with the chopped scallions.

PROTEIN DRINKS

The base for these delicious protein drinks is seeds and nuts, which are a source of excellent protein. Seeds and nuts also contain protease inhibitors, protective factors that have anti–aging benefits and may help prevent cancer. These drinks are a delicious alternative to dairy products for a protein–rich beverage. Soaking the nuts and seeds overnight before blending them enhances their digestibility and triggers the release of the nutrients.

Helpful Hints

* These protein drinks can be refrigerated for a full 24 hours, but it is best to make them daily and use them as soon as possible to derive their nutritional value.

* Fill a thermos and bring it to work for a midmorning or midafternoon snack.

* These drinks are protein–rich, so be sure to wait at least two hours after your fruit breakfast before using a protein drink as a midmorning snack.

* If you find that you like to have two protein drinks a day, double the recipes.

Almond Milk
(Yields 3 cups)

1/2 cup almonds
purified water to soak almonds
3 cups purified water
1 tablespoon honey
pinch of sea salt
1 teaspoon sesame oil

1. Soak the almonds overnight in enough purified water to cover.

2. In the morning, pour off and discard the soak water. Slip the skins off the almonds with a gentle squeeze.

3. Place the almonds, 3 cups of purified water, honey, sea salt, and sesame oil in a blender and blend. If desired, you may strain the drink through a cheesecloth. (I like the crunchiness of the unstrained drink. If you do not strain it, be sure to chew your drink well!).

Sesame–Seed Milk
(Yields 3 cups)

1/2 cup sesame seeds
3 cups purified water

---

1 tablespoon rice syrup or honey

1. Grind the seeds in a coffee grinder or blender.
2. Blend all of the ingredients in a blender.
3. Strain the hulls through a strainer or cheesecloth.

Sunflower–Seed Milk
(Yields 3 cups)

1/3 cup sunflower seeds, hulled and unsalted
purified water to soak sunflower seeds
3 cups purified water
1 tablespoon rice syrup, if desired

1. Soak the seeds overnight in enough purified water to cover.

2. Pour off and discard the soak water. Place the soaked seeds and 3 cups of water in a blender and blend.

3. This mixture is sweeter than the Almond Milk and Sesame–Seed Milk, but you may add 1 tablespoon of rice syrup or honey if you wish.

The following four protein drinks use the first three recipes as a base. Each of these recipes makes one serving.

Hot Mock Chocolate
(Serves 1)

---

1 tablespoon carob powder
1 tablespoon honey
1 cup nut or seed milk

1. Add the carob powder and honey to one cup of any of the nut or seed milks.

2. Warm the mixture and drink it immediately, or store it in a thermos for later use.

Maple–Nut Shake
(Serves 1)

---

1 tablespoon almond butter
1 teaspoon pure maple syrup
1 cup Almond Milk

Place all the ingredients in a blender and blend thoroughly.

Tahini Shake
(Serves 1)

---

1 tablespoon tahini
1 teaspoon honey
1 cup Sesame–Seed Milk

Place all the ingredients in a blender and blend thoroughly.

Carrot Shake
(Serves 1)

---

4 ounces fresh carrot juice
4 ounces Sesame–Seed Milk

Place the carrot juice and the Sesame–Seed Milk in a blender and blend.

Variations

* For a different flavor, try the Almond or Sunflower–Seed Milk in place of the Sesame–Seed Milk.

CLEANSING JUICE BLENDS

Use only fresh-squeezed juices from raw organic vegetables, or the vegetables that you have treated with the Cleansing Soak for Fruits and Vegetables on page 88.

CONSTIPATION CURE: Six ounces carrot juice and two ounces spinach juice.

BLOOD BUILDER: Six ounces carrot juice, one ounce beet juice, and one ounce parsley or watercress juice.

COMPLEXION TONIC: Three ounces carrot juice, three ounces cucumber juice, and two ounces beet juice.

BREATH FRESHENER: Two ounces of any combination of: parsley, spinach, watercress, comfrey, and alfalfa juices; and three ounces carrot juice and three ounces celery juice.

CALMING COCKTAIL: Five ounces carrot juice and three ounces celery juice.

DIGESTIVE TONER: Four ounces of carrot juice and four ounces cabbage juice.

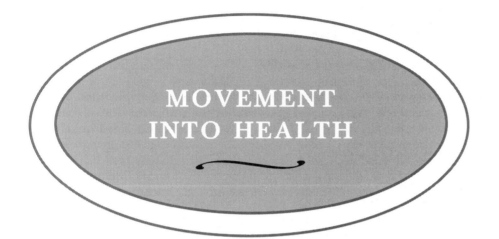

MOVEMENT INTO HEALTH

*D*oing exercise that you enjoy is a key to your Cleansing and Rejuvenation Program. I remember that when I was younger, exercise was practically my whole life. I spent much of my time dancing, swimming, riding my bicycle, and enjoying the exuberant energy and freedom of youth. I never thought of these activities as work; they were my greatest source of pleasure. As I grew older and became busy with my studies and my career, I became more sedentary. For years I got very little exercise. I was lucky that I was able to maintain the tone I had developed when I was younger because I was getting regular massage.

Finally, as I neared thirty, my health and appearance became more important concerns for me, and I realized I needed to set up an exercise program. I tried jogging and exercise classes, but somehow they seemed more a chore than a pleasure. When I injured my knee while running, my doctor suggested I take up swimming. Suddenly, I rediscovered the joy I had felt as a young swimmer, when exercise was so natural for me. I got myself a new bicycle, and I still ride it to my office whenever possible. In addition, I started walking regularly and continued swimming once a week. I began to realize that all the activities I had enjoyed years ago were exercise, and I simply put them back into my life.

BRISK–PACE WALKING

A central feature of your 21–Day Program is an invigorating daily walk outdoors. Walking is a natural function of the human body. It provides all the benefits of other forms of vigorous exercise. It is easy, it requires no special equipment, and, as you will see for yourself, it is enjoyable.

Walking has become an essential part of my lifestyle. Living in the lovely town of Sausalito, California, I have endless opportunities for walks in nature, enjoying the views and the fresh air along San Francisco Bay. An early morning walk, with a stop for tea at my favorite cafe, is one of my most treasured rituals.

Of course, it takes some discipline to develop a daily practice of aerobic activity, which takes walking one step further. People who exercise regularly can tell you that it makes them feel great, and years of medical research have verified the benefits. Exercise has powerful psychological effects. It alleviates anxiety, elevates the mood, and produces an enhanced sense of well–being. Exercise also promotes the inner and outer cleansing that is the goal of this program. The increased intake of oxygen during exercise accelerates the burning of wastes that otherwise accumulate in the tissues and joints. Brisk movement promotes the circulation of blood, carrying nutrients to the tissues and removing toxins, and it stimulates the flow of lymph to carry away debris. Increased perspiration during exercise eliminates wastes through the skin. Exercise also stimulates the function of the internal organs and intestines, promoting better digestion and elimination.

INNER CLEANSING THROUGH EXERCISE

Active people who walk as part of their regular routine are much less likely to suffer from heart disease, high blood pressure, and other afflictions of our high–tech lifestyle. Exercise helps to control cholesterol levels, preventing the formation of plaque deposits in the arteries. Physical activity, especially exercise that makes the bones bear the body's weight, such as walking, also helps to build up the mineral content in the bones, protecting against osteoporosis, the loss of bone mass that has become such a problem among older people, especially women.

Brisk walking is one of the most important keys to maintaining a youthful appearance. It promotes clear skin and healthy color, and is a crucial factor in weight control. People who do one hour of energetic walking each day can generally eat just about anything they want without gaining weight. Not only does the walking itself burn calories and body fat, it also helps to decrease appetite.

Scientists who have studied the legendary isolated groups of people who remain healthy into their eighties and nineties and over, have found that regular exercise is one of the key factors contributing to their longevity. The Hunza of Pakistan and the Vilcabamba of Ecuador, for example, walk up and down their native mountains as part of their daily activity. Exercise also promotes longevity by enhancing one's sense of well–being. And this positive mental state is another of the important keys to a healthy and vital long life.

To derive the greatest benefit from brisk walking, you must provide your body with the proper nutrients to supply energy and build new cells. Especially important is the mineral potassium, which is often deficient in our overly sodium–laden diet. Potassium supports proper muscle tone. Remember, the heart and intestines have muscle tissue. Low tissue–potassium levels can lead to muscle spasm and fatigue; such muscle problems are frequently an underlying cause of low back discomfort and even constipation.

Many of the soups and bisques I recommend in the Body–Smart Recipes, on pages 94 through 97 are based on my mineral–rich Potassium Broth—one of the essential liquid foods of the Clean and Clear Diet. Potassium Broth provides important minerals to help keep your cells and muscles properly nourished as you go in and out of the fast in the second and third weeks of the program.

Because you perspire during vigorous activity, your body needs extra fluid to support an exercise program. I recommend drinking plenty of fluids before and after exercise, but not during the actual exercise period. For a walk of one–half hour, there's no need to carry water with you. Drink the Oxygenation Cocktail on page 82 just before exercising each day for a powerful cleansing and rejuvenating effect.

MAKING YOUR WORKOUT WORK FOR YOU

A strong heart and healthy lungs are central to any cleansing and fitness program. The stronger your heart is, the less work it will have to do to pump blood, nutrients, and oxygen to all the tissues in your body. When your heart is in good condition, it beats harder but less frequently.

The best kind of exercise to keep your heart and lungs in top condition is aerobic, which means "with oxygen." Through continuous, vigorous movements of the large muscles, you are speeding up your heartbeat and breathing more deeply, sending a richer supply of oxygen to nourish your tissues.

When you are exercising aerobically, you will feel your heart beating faster, and your breathing will speed up. As your body heats up, your skin becomes moist, and after a while you begin to feel exhilarated. After an aerobic workout, you will feel a glow and sense of well–being that will last for hours.

Brisk walking allows you to enjoy the well–publicized benefits of aerobic exercise in a way that is safe and gentle to your bones, joints, and muscles. I know that many joggers have injured their feet, ankles, knees or backs with the high impact and stress of their chosen sport. If you truly enjoy jogging then keep it up; but please be sure always to do warm–up exercises before you jog, and cool–down activities afterward, to minimize the chance of injury. In addition, try to jog on dirt trails or on sand, since jogging on cement or asphalt jars the lower body.

Other forms of exercise besides walking also provide safe aerobic conditioning. Swimming is a wonderful alternative, which we will explore on page 125. Many people like bicycling and find it a much better way to get around than in their cars. Dancing is a lively activity that you can do in public places, in aerobics classes, or at home by simply putting on some of your favorite music. Skiing, especially cross–country skiing, provides an excellent workout if you have access to snow and equipment. The main criterion is that you select an exercise that you enjoy, because that is the best guarantee that you will keep it up. Vary your choice of exercise to suit your mood, your schedule, or the season.

Use the Oxygen Consumption During Exercise chart on page 119, to compare the relative strenuousness of various popular forms of exercise. The figures represent calories burned, but were actually determined by measuring the amount of oxygen consumed—that is, how aerobic the exercise is.

As you get in better shape, you will need to exercise more vigorously to derive the same benefits. That is the time to add more exertion to your workout. It always takes effort to enjoy the rewards of exercise, but you will soon learn that such exertion can be very worthwhile.

The experience of one of my clients, Monica, is a good example of the dramatic benefits of stepping up the challenge of an exercise program. I had been working with Monica on a cleansing and weight–loss program for about five months. She had been losing weight steadily and was looking radiant from the cleansing, but she had gotten to the point where the weight just wasn't coming off quickly enough. Every time she came in, I would ask her whether she had been exercising, and she would say "yes". Finally, I asked what kind of exercise she had been doing, and she told me she had been taking a nice, leisurely walk for about forty–five minutes every day. "That may have been enough a few months ago," I said, "but now you need to include more aerobic activity in your walk." I encouraged her to push herself just beyond her comfort level, that point where she wanted to stop. Since Monica lived in San Francisco, she began walking briskly up and down the hills, instead of on level ground. When she came in two weeks later, I was amazed at how much weight she had lost. She was spending the same amount of time on her exercise, but because she was getting more aerobic activity from hill–walking, she had given her metabolism a boost, and the weight was coming off very quickly again.

Just as important as committing yourself to a daily exercise program is developing an exercise attitude. Get into the habit of walking to work or to the store. If you use public transportation, get off a few blocks away from your destination and walk the rest of the way. Use stairs instead of elevators or escalators. When you feel groggy or bored, take a short, brisk walk instead of a snack or a cup of coffee. By making exercise a natural, joyful part of your life, you will guarantee yourself added years of vibrant beauty and good health.

BUILDING A LIFETIME WALKING HABIT

The hardest part of any exercise program is actually getting started. Since it takes about three weeks to establish a new habit, your 21–Day Program is an ideal beginning. As you begin to feel the elation and increased vigor that are immediate benefits of regular brisk walking, you will become more and more motivated to keep it up. Eventually, when you experience the long–term benefits, you will most likely become a lifelong walker.

In the Self–Assessment Questionnaire on pages 13 through 21 and Setting Your Goals on pages 25 through 30, you evaluated your level of fitness, established your goals, and constructed your exercise schedule. Begin an Exercise Log in your journal and use it each day to record your daily work-out. Over the course of your three–week program, you will see an improvement in your stamina and conditioning, as indicated by an increase in the speed, distance, or time you record in your Exercise Log. Just as I encouraged Monica to push herself beyond the point of wanting to stop, I encourage you to do the same, just a bit farther each day! I recommend about one-half hour of brisk walking every day. If you have been telling yourself up until now that you just don't have the time to spend on regular exercise, get up a half hour earlier, and do your walking then. At the end of your exercise period, ask yourself if it was worth it. Your sense of well–being and the glow in your body will tell you that it was.

Since walking is such a safe activity, most people will be able to begin their walking program immediately. If you are over forty–five and are not now exercising regularly, you should consult a physician before beginning any exercise program. If you have high blood pressure, heart disease, or other problems requiring medical attention, no matter what your age, you should also check with your doctor. Most likely you will get an enthusiastic go–ahead.

One of the nicest things about walking is that you don't need any special equipment. Of course, you do need to wear comfortable, sturdy shoes, but please don't fall victim to the notion that you must have a different pair of shoes for every activity. Running shoes, lightweight hiking boots, or tennis shoes are fine. Specially designed walking shoes are heavier than running shoes but lighter than regular shoes, making it easier to lift your feet. What-ever shoes you wear, make sure they are a comfortable fit, leaving enough room to wiggle your toes, and that they are flexible enough to allow for nor-mal walking motion. The shoes should allow your feet to breathe; leather, canvas, or nylon mesh, or combinations of these, are suitable materials. The shoes should have thick, flexible soles to absorb shock, and cushioned insoles to help prevent blisters. Wear cotton socks to allow your feet to breathe and perspire freely.

When you walk, wear comfortable, loose-fitting clothing of natural fibers so that your skin can breathe, too. You may want to layer your clothing so you can remove the outer layer as you warm up. If you are walking on sunny days, wear a hat to protect your face from harmful ultraviolet rays, and do use a unblock, even when it is overcast. To allow your arms to swing freely when you walk, you may want to use a waist pack or a small day pack if you need to carry anything with you.

Part of the fun of walking is the opportunity it provides to be out in nature. America's great naturalist Henry David Thoreau wrote, "I think that I can-not preserve my health and spirits unless I spend four hours a day at least—and it is commonly more than that—sauntering through the woods and over the hills and fields, absolutely free from all worldly engagements." Today's busy lifestyles do not permit most of us to walk for four hours a day in nature, but you can experience some of the same benefits on shorter walks if you select a route that exposes you to plenty of fresh air, greenery, or water.

Take a moment now to think about the opportunities for walking in your community. Do you live near an ocean, a river, a reservoir, or a lake? The air near running water or breaking waves is rich in negative ions, which increase your alertness and sense of optimism. Perhaps there are woods or open fields near your home. Every city has parks. You might select a route that takes you from your home to the nearest park, through the park and back. Another possibility would be to drive or bike to a park, do your walking there, and then ride back. Or take a bus to some distant location close to nature and walk home. Choose a route that allows you to walk two to three miles. Even if you don't walk that far at first, you will eventually build up to that distance.

It is a fact of modern life that many of us live in crowded, noisy urban areas. If you simply cannot get away from city streets and sidewalks, I suggest that you use a portable cassette player and listen to your favorite music. Try to avoid streets where traffic produces smoggy air.

People differ in their preferences about when to do their walking. In general, the best time to exercise is before eating. Brisk walking before meals produces a rise in blood sugar that will decrease your appetite and boost your metabolic rate. Many people find that going for a walk first thing in the morning gives them a burst of energy and a positive mental attitude that carries them through the day. Others find that vigorous exercise after a day of work helps them to unwind and relax. Some people prefer to use a portion of their lunchtime for a brisk walk to help break up the stress of the workday. Whatever time of day you choose, remember that your exercise period is a gift to yourself, a time to enjoy the pleasure of movement and being out of doors—to free yourself, like Thoreau, from "all worldly engagements."

WARMING UP AND COOLING DOWN

Even for low–impact exercise like walking, it is important to do warm–up exercises before you begin. Warming up prepares your body by stimulating the flow of blood and oxygen to the heart. It warms the muscles so they become more elastic and are less likely to be injured. Here are several warm–ups you may use throughout my program before your daily exercise. Each warm–up is a series of movements and stretches, many of which are based on yoga. The postures of hatha yoga are scientifically designed to promote rejuvenation and regeneration by stimulating and regulating the endocrine glands that govern the aging process. These are not calisthenics. Do not move quickly from one part of the activity to the next, but take the time to relax after each phase and feel its benefits.

Wake–up Shake–up

This is a favorite moving meditation of mine. It is a great way to warm up the muscles, enhance your body awareness, and release emotional tension.

Stand relaxed with your feet apart and parallel to each other. Imagine that the balls of your feet are glued to the floor. Begin to wake up your body by slowly and rhythmically lifting your hells, one foot and then the other, while keeping the balls of your feet on the floor. Imagine you are walking without lifting your feet. After lifting alternate heels for a while, begin to include your legs. Keep the balls of your feet in place on the floor with your knees slightly bent, pretending you are walking but keeping your feet in place. Next, rhythmically move to include your knees. Now, begin to shake your legs all the way from the ankles to the hips, with the balls of your feet still planted on the floor. Wake up the whole bottom of your body. Shake your legs, your buttocks, gradually moving the shaking all the way up your body. Shake your shoulders, arms, and hands. Loosen up, shaking all over. Stop, relax for a moment, and feel the effects throughout your entire being.

Now, raise your arms over your head. Stretch from the waist up, and feel the pull from the waist down. Allow your body to hang for a minute or so. Breathe in as you raise your arms above your head, then slowly and gently exhale, bending down toward the floor, keeping your knees loose and relaxed. Breathe rhythmically throughout this exercise. Do not hold your breath. After you have awakened your whole body with this shake and stretch, begin your day's exercise.

Dancer's Warm-up

These isolated movements of different body parts are warm-ups from an Afro-Haitian dance class that I attended for years, and many of them have their roots in yoga. Dancers know that they have to warm up every part of the body before they can do any more strenuous dance routines. Warm-up activity is probably 50 percent of every dance class. You may wish to read this routine into your tape recorder so that you can play it back before your daily walks.

Begin with neck rolls. Bring your left ear down to your left shoulder, roll your neck all the way to the back, over to the right shoulder, and then down so your chin touches your chest. Keep the neck moving, using a continuous, smooth, rolling movement. Repeat five times, then reverse direction and roll your neck five times in the opposite direction. Breathe in as you roll your neck back, and breathe out as you roll your neck forward.

Next, do shoulder rolls. Rotate your left shoulder backward five times, then forward five times. Repeat for the right shoulder. Then roll both shoulders together, five times backward and five times forward. Continue the breathing pattern you established with the neck rolls.

Follow with a spinal twist. Stand relaxed with your feet apart at about shoulder width. Keep your lower body in position and twist from the waist up, bringing your torso all the way around to the left, as you are trying to touch the back of your waist with your right hand. Twist all the way around, looking as far behind you as you can over your left shoulder. Now, holding this position, turn your head around and look as far as you can to the right to provide a full-body stretch. Return to a relaxed center position and reverse direction, twisting your torso to the right. Repeat each direction five time. Breathe in as you move to the left, and breathe out as you twist to the right.

With your feet still apart at shoulder distance, extend your arms in front of you at shoulder level and do some gentle knee bends. Move slowly, avoiding any bouncing movements. Don't be alarmed if your knees creak. Repeat five times, breathing out as you lower yourself and in as you rise.

Now, lift one foot at a time and rotate the ankle, twisting each foot clockwise and then counterclockwise, wiggling your toes and tightening and releasing the arches of your feet. Repeat five times for each foot, maintaining your breathing pattern as you go.

End with a good upward stretch. Breathe in, extending your arms over your head. Breathe out and bend down to touch the floor. Relax and hang for a few moments, breathing normally.

In addition to warming up, allow time at the end of your daily exercise for cool–down activity. Without gentle movement at the end of a workout, the blood remains pooled out in the arms and legs; as a result, you may experience dizziness and nausea. An easy way to cool down after walking or running is to slacken your pace to a slow walk for about five minutes.

LYMPH CLEANSING WARM–UP

You will perform the Lymph Cleansing Warm–up every day during Week 2 or whenever you wish, in order to pump the lymph forcefully through your body. Vigorous movement of the arms and legs aids in cleansing the system by encouraging waste–laden lymph to be carried away from the cells for elimination. The warm–up will take about twelve minutes. It is fun to do to music.

MARCHING IN PLACE. Begin by marching briskly in place. Lift your knees in an exaggerated marching step. As you lift one leg, swing the opposite arm forward, and swing the arm on the same side as far back as it can go. Keep your arms straight but relaxed as you swing them vigorously back and forth from the shoulders. Keep your spine straight and your head high. Continue for about three minutes to really get the lymph moving. Then stop and rest in the standing position for a moment, feeling the effects of this brisk exercise.

ALTERNATE ARM RAISES. Lie on your back on the floor with your arms at your sides and your knees up, with the feet slightly separated. Raise one arm up and back so that it rests on the floor behind your head. Now, return this arm to its original position at your side, while you raise the other arm and let it rest on the floor behind your head. Keeping your arms straight, continue this alternating movement fairly rapidly, about one second for each arm raise. Breathe in as you raise one arm, and out as you raise the other. Continue for about three minutes, then relax with both arms at your sides and feel the effects of the pumping movement.

SIDE LEG LIFTS. Lie on your right side with your legs straight and your head cradled on your right arm. Lift your left leg sideways, up toward the ceiling, keeping your toes turned in, pigeon–toed. Go slowly, stretching your leg up sideways as much as possible; take about two seconds to raise the leg and two to lower it. Continue for about two minutes, then repeat while lying on the left side. End by relaxing flat on your back for a few minutes in the resting pose. Breathe normally, feeling the stimulating effects of the leg movements.

Oxygen Consumption During Exercise

(Expressed as calories burned per minute)

ACTIVITY	WEIGHT IN POUNDS			
	100–119	120–144	145–174	175–200
BICYCLING				
leisurely	3.16	3.58	4.25	4.66
moderate	5.41	6.16	7.33	7.91
brisk	8.58	9.75	11.50	12.66
DANCING				
aerobic	5.83	6.58	7.83	8.58
rock	3.25	3.75	4.41	4.91
GARDENING				
weeding and digging	5.08	5.75	6.83	7.50
JOGGING				
5.5 mph	8.58	9.75	11.50	12.66
6.5 mph	8.90	10.20	12.00	13.20
8.0 mph	10.40	11.90	14.10	15.50
9.0 mph	12.00	13.80	16.20	17.80
SEXUAL INTERCOURSE				
active partner	3.91	4.50	5.25	5.83
SKIING				
downhill	7.75	8.83	10.41	11.50
cross-country, moderate	9.16	10.41	12.25	13.33
cross-country, brisk	13.08	14.83	17.58	19.33
STAIR-CLIMBING				
normal	5.90	6.70	7.90	8.80
upstairs rapidly	8.70	14.80	17.60	19.30
SWIMMING				
leisurely	3.91	4.50	5.25	5.83
moderate	7.83	8.91	10.50	11.58
brisk	11.00	12.50	14.75	16.25
TENNIS				
singles	7.83	8.91	10.50	11.58
doubles	5.58	6.33	7.50	8.25
WALKING				
leisurely	2.40	2.80	3.30	3.60
moderate	3.90	4.50	5.30	5.80
brisk	4.50	5.20	6.10	6.80

WALKING-ENHANCEMENT TECHNIQUES

It may seem unnecessary to have instructions for such a natural activity as walking, but the more aware you are of your body and your surroundings, the more benefit you will derive from your daily walks. Join me now, as I guide you through an easy, enjoyable walk that will give you a mental lift, condition your muscles, and carry oxygen to all the cells of your body.

Before you begin walking, take a moment to pay attention to posture. Nothing can age your appearance more quickly than poor body alignment. Your spine is one of the most important parts of your body; when it is not properly aligned, your internal organs cannot work as effectively.

For a quick posture check, imagine you are balancing a heavy basket on your head. Pull up, and feel your spine straighten.

Now, begin with five minutes of slow, gentle walking. Swing your arms freely at your sides, use a heel–to–toe gait, and keep your posture in mind. Gradually increase your pace until you are walking briskly. Swing your arms quite strongly at right angles, back and forward, to stimulate the flow of lymph. For most adults, a pace of three to four miles per hour will provide the same aerobic conditioning benefits as jogging or other vigorous activities. Notice how your breathing and heartbeat speed up.

Keep up your rapid aerobic pace for twelve to fifteen minutes, and preferably longer. At the end of the brisk walking period, return to a slow pace for five minutes to allow your body to cool down.

As you walk, pay attention to your breathing and establish a comfortable rhythm. Count along with the beat of each step, practicing the following breathing patterns as part of your regular walking exercise.

Meditative Walking Breath

Breathing patterns derived from yoga can help to bring your body, mind, and spirit into harmony as you walk. Nothing helps you center yourself better than focusing on your breath.

Breathe in through both nostrils to the count of four paces. Hold your breath in for a count of four, then breathe out through pursed lips to a count of four. Repeat the cycle; in to four, hold for four, and out to four, as you walk along briskly. This 4–4–4 breath is wonderfully invigorating.

As you breathe, be aware of your surroundings. Feel the cool, clean air enter your lungs. Notice the fresh, natural smells around you, the aroma of trees or water. Breathing in to the count of four, inhale the sights, smells, and sounds of nature. Open your hands and feel the green of the trees, the blue of the sky, the warmth of the sun. Then, for the next four paces, hold your breath and feel the glow throughout your body, the warmth and tingle in your arms and legs. With each step, be aware of the movement of the bones and muscles in your feet. Now, breathe out on the next four paces, and as you breathe out, release all the negative thoughts that flit through your mind. Let go of your anxieties and worries, and feel the toxins being released from your body, the waste products being expelled through your breath and sweat. Breathe in to the count of four and focus on positive thoughts: peace,

REBOUNDING WORKOUT

One of the best forms of exercise for stimulating the lymph system is rebounding on a mini trampoline. Rebounding stimulates lymphatic circulation because it produces a change in the body's fluid pressure with relatively little muscular effort. At the bottom of each bounce, waste products and toxins are squeezed out from between the cells. When the body rebounds into the air, nutrients pass from the lymph into the cells. At the height of the bounce, the body is weightless, and the lymph begins to flow. As the body descends, the lymphatic fluid flows along, pulling the extracted wastes along with it.

Rebounding has all the benefits of aerobic exercise, but it does not jar the skeletal system the way some exercises do. You can buy a reasonably priced mini trampoline at most sporting goods stores. I highly recommend this piece of equipment as part of your exercise program. There are many different exercises you can do–to music, or while watching television–that make this an easy and pleasurable way to maintain your aerobic conditioning and stimulate and cleanse your lymph system.

harmony, joy, well-being. Find the words that seem best for you, and breathe them in with each inhalation. Hold for the count of four and feel the glow. Exhale to the count of four and release, relax, and be at peace with yourself.

Once you have mastered the 4-4-4 breath, vary your breathing pattern by inhaling to the count of six, holding the breath in for three, exhaling for six counts, and holding the breath out for three, with the lungs empty of air. Then repeat the 6-3-6-3 pattern. This breathing pattern helps dispel tension and anxiety whenever you feel it creeping up on you during the day. Use it regularly on your walks, or at any other time you want to relax and unwind.

A further variation you can try is an 8-4-8-4 breath, inhaling for eight counts, holding the breath for four, exhaling for eight, and holding the breath out for four. I find this pattern even more calming than the 6-3-6-3. Besides using it with walking, try it when you are upset or are having difficulty getting to sleep.

If you regularly practice these breathing patterns and the sensory awareness that goes with them, they will become a habit. You will be inhaling peace, serenity, and joy, and exhaling all your worries, whenever you walk.

At the end of your daily walk, be aware of how you feel. Ask yourself, do I feel less tired than when I started? Am I in a better mood? Do I feel more relaxed? Each time you check in with your mind and body at the end of an exercise period and recognize the positive benefits, you are giving yourself additional reinforcement for the next workout.

EXERCISE FOR LIFE

Research has shown that people who continue their exercise program for twenty weeks are likely to continue exercising all their lives. At that point, their self-esteem improves dramatically, and exercise then becomes self-reinforcing. Do not hesitate to try variations in your exercise activities to keep up your interest and motivation. Above all, remember always to do exercise that you enjoy.

Over time, you will need to exercise more vigorously to enjoy the same health benefits, since your muscles will become stronger and will not have to work as hard. To make your exercise more challenging, try walking briskly uphill, or hold your arms out at a ninety-degree angle and pump them energetically as you walk. Alternate between skipping five minutes, then walking five minutes; marching five minutes, swinging your arms briskly at your sides with your posture straight and tall, then walking five minutes. You may also alternate five minutes of walking with five minutes of jogging, if you wish, but be sure you are well warmed up before you begin to jog.

Just as you vary your exercise activities, vary the setting. Find several different routes that you enjoy. Change your activity as the seasons change, or try walking before dawn, after sunset, or in the rain, for a different sensory experience. If you usually walk alone, try walking with a partner, or form a walking group to give each other mutual support. If you have a dog, it will be delighted to romp along with you at your fastest pace. If you have children, get them to establish a walking habit with you. They may not be able to keep up with your rapid aerobic pace or to walk as long as you do, so you might spend half an hour doing brisk walking at one time during the day, and then join your kids for another short walk later. Walking with children in nature is a wonderful opportunity for learning. Talk about what you see. Point out and name the trees, birds, and flowers. They will probably have something to teach you, too.

RESISTANCE TONING FOR SUPPLE MUSCLES

Aerobic activity is not the only form of exercise you need. Especially if one of your goals on this program is to lose weight, you will benefit from the toning that comes from resistance training, or using your muscles against the force of gravity. I work out regularly with small dumbbells at home to strengthen and tone my upper body. The free weights let me make adjustments in muscle motion angles that are not possible with exercise machines.

Besides the muscle toning that resistance training provides, it also helps to send oxygen–bearing blood into parts of the body that are difficult to reach with your breath and puts oxygen deep into the tissues. It also provides an opportunity to direct your full attention to the specific part of the body that you want to strengthen and fill with oxygen.

ANTI–GRAVITY TONE–UP

The slant board has long been a beauty secret of health–conscious people. It works by reversing the effects of gravity. The aging process causes the skin, facial features, and internal organs to droop. When you lie with your head below your feet, the effects of gravity are reversed, and all the organs are in a relaxed, suspended position. Blood flows to the face, neck, and head, bringing nutrients and oxygen to the brain and facial tissues and improving the complexion. The antigravity position on the slant board relieves sinus problems and eyestrain and helps to eliminate wrinkles. It improves circulation throughout the body, and is very helpful for anyone with distressed organs. A few minutes on a slant board in the antigravity position provides a quick pick–me–up, revitalizing your brain cells and restoring your energy. (If you have high blood pressure or other medical problems, check with your doctor before using a slant board. Except for specific cautions, daily use of a slant board will generally help any health problem.)

If you don't have a slant board, you can make your own by covering a board with padding and securely tacking it down. The board should be longer than you are tall and at least as wide as your body when your arms are at your side. Rest the slant board on a stable surface so it is at an angle of twenty to forty–five degrees, then lie on it with your feet up and your head down. If you cannot find a board the right size, try improvising with an ironing board so you can begin to experience the benefits of the Anti–gravity Tone–up.

The following activities will help to improve both your strength and your appearance. Again, you may wish to read these exercises into your tape recorder and create a routine for repetitions.

Beauty Exercise

Lying on your back on the slant board, exhale all the breath from your lungs. Touch your lower waist with your fingertips while exhaling, and see how small you can get your waist to be. Keeping your lungs deflated, draw your chest toward your chin, tensing the abdominal muscles at the same time. Draw your waist in, as small as you can. Pull everything in and up inside. Then relax and breathe normally. This is another exercise derived from yoga. It will help slim your waist and get rid of fatty deposits around your middle. Repeat the exercise ten times, then relax in a resting pose on the slant board, in the antigravity position.

Alternate Knee Lifts

These knee lifts will begin to tone and strengthen your abdominal muscles in preparation for more challenging exercises later. Bring one knee up to the chest, inhaling as you do so. As you exhale, straighten and lower that leg and simultaneously bring the other bent knee up. Keep the toes pointed, and the straightened legs parallel to the slant board; you are not trying to pedal high in the air. Breathe in as you lift one knee, and out as you lift the other, maintaining a brisk pace. Start by doing ten lifts for each knee, increasing gradually over time until you can do thirty. After the exercise, relax in the resting position.

Palming

Finish your Antigravity Tone–up with this pleasant facial muscle relaxer and eye revitalizer. Rub your palms together until you feel the heat. Then cup your hands over your closed eyes, crossing your fingertips over your forehead. Be sure to cover your eyes completely, so no light would get in even if your eyes were open. Feel the heat going into your closed eyes, and the relaxation spreading to all the muscles of your face. Let go of the tension in your jaw, lips, and cheeks, and let the relaxation spread down to your neck and throat, out to your shoulders, and down your arms. Relax your back, chest, rib cage, abdomen, hops, and thighs, your lower legs, feet, and hands. Often tension accumulates in the eyes. As you release this tension, you not only renew and beautify your eyes but allow the relaxation to spread to every part of your body. Stay with this at least five minutes.

REVITALIZATION THROUGH YOGA

Yoga has been done throughout the world for centuries and is known to maintain youthful attitudes, appearance, mobility, and organ health. Western cultures tend to benefit from the stress reduction benefits as well. Many people I have known who have practiced yoga throughout their lives have maintained a glowing youthful vitality far beyond those who have not.

Yoga activates areas along the spine, directing nourishing blood and nerve impulses to the body's organs. It helps to wake up the joints and connective tissue and improves the circulation of both blood and lymph. Specific postures target specific organs, joints, and other areas of the body. The gentle stretching movements of yoga help to stimulate areas that are difficult to reach.

YOGA ARCH POSE VARIATIONS

The Yoga Arch Pose and its variations are excellent toners of the entire abdominal region. The pose helps to promote digestion and is also very relaxing. Lie on your back on the floor, with your arms resting at your sides. Bring your knees up to a bent position with the feet side by side. Push off your body from the floor with your hips, keeping your knees bent. Bring the pelvis up in the air and arch the back, so that your body forms an arch supported by the back of your neck and shoulders, and your feet. Hold this position for as long as is comfortable, then lower your pelvis to the floor and relax. Then go up again, this time arching your back even higher. Come down and rest once again. Now, lift the pelvis again, and this time while you are up, tense your whole body and then relax it, tense it and relax it, finally lowering the pelvis to the floor and resting. Go up again, repeat the tensing and relaxing two or three times, then come down and rest. Finally, raise the pelvis again, and this time as you remain in the arch position, pull the abdominal muscles in and up, giving your abdominal organs an internal massage as you pull in and narrow your waist. Lower your pelvis to the floor and relax, breathing naturally for a few minutes.

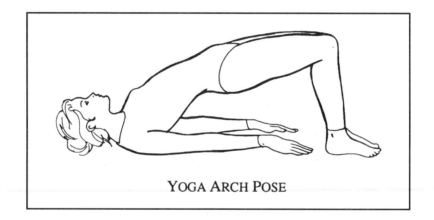

YOGA ARCH POSE

Perform each of the variations on the Arch Pose as many times as you wish. You will find it is very stimulating to the abdominal organs, and it leaves you with a wonderful relaxed feeling.

YOGA STRESS RELEASERS

Before you begin this exercise, you may wish to read it slowly into a tape recorder. This way you can play it back, instructing yourself, without breaking your concentration to refer to the book.

Lie quietly on your back on the floor, with your arms at your sides and your heels lightly touching. Relax for a moment with your eyes closed and breath normally. Now, raise your hands and feet straight up in the air. Hold them that way for a few moments, and then begin to shake your arms and legs, your hands and feet. Shake them vigorously, feeling them loosen up, shaking out all the stress. Let go of all the tension in your muscles. Let your hands and feet flop back and forth at the ends of your arms and legs. Con-

> ### YOGIC SWIMMING
>
> Swimming is one of the best exercises for developing your breathing capacity. It uses all the muscles of the body, and the motion of the arms helps to develop the cartilage between the ribs, aiding in chest expansion. When done correctly, swimming is not strenuous. It has a relaxing effect on the nerves and stimulates circulation. As you glide through the water, all your tissues and organs receive a gentle, invigorating hydromassage.
>
> The crawl is especially good for deep breathing. Experiment with variations in your breathing pattern. Instead of breathing on every other stroke so that you always breathe to the same side, try breathing on every third stroke, so that you breathe alternately to the left and the right. This helps to balance your nervous-system function and keeps you more aware of your breathing.
>
> Use your swimming time as an opportunity to experience the relaxing effects of breath. Focus on positive thoughts as you breathe in, and exhale anxiety and stress. Keep your attention on your breath; get into the rhythm of its ebb and flow, and you will move into a blissful state that goes with the peaceful energy of effortless, gliding movement.
>
> Swim continuously for at least twelve minutes to achieve aerobic benefits, with the eventual goal of building up to swimming without stopping for twenty minutes. If you don't swim for the full twenty minutes, enjoy some of your time simply floating, breathing, stretching, and relaxing as your body is supported by the water.

tinue this shaking for a few minutes, then return your arms and legs to the resting position and feel the effects of releasing the tension.

Next, in the lying position, I want you to go through each part of your body, tensing and releasing. This exercise is designed to let you experience the greatest tension you can feel, before you release it and let it go. Lie quietly with your eyes closed, breathing gently. Now, bring your attention to your feet. Breathe in through the nostrils, and tense both feet, as tense as you can get them. When you feel the greatest tension you are capable of feeling, breathe out through pursed lips, and as you release your breath, release the tension from your feet. Relax and breathe normally for a moment, feeling the effects of this release.

Now, as you inhale, begin to tense again, not only the feet but also the calves. Tense as much as you can, and as you release your breath, let go of the tension, first from the calves and then the feet. Feel the tension not just in the muscles, but also in the nerves, the blood vessels, and even the bones.

Again breathe in through the nostrils, tense the feet and the calves, then add the thighs and hips. As you release your breath through pursed lips, release the tension downward, from the hips and thighs to the calves and feet. Relax for a moment and enjoy the feeling of releasing the tension.

Now, breathe in again, and tense upward from the feet to the thighs and hips, and now add the abdominal section and lower back. Feel the internal abdominal organs tensing and contracting, so that you are completely tensed from the waist down. As you release your breath, first let go in the abdomen.

Feel the abdominal organs relax, then release the tension downward, ending with the feet. Each time, release more deeply than the time before. On the next inhalation, tense upward to the abdomen, and now add the upper torso, the chest, back, and spine. Feel everything completely and evenly tightened and tense. Release your breath, and let go of the tension first in the chest, down the spine, into the abdomen, and down to the feet.

Breathe in, tense from the feet up through the upper torso, and now make a fist with your hands, tensing up the arms into the shoulders. As you exhale, release the arms and hands, moving down all the way to the feet.

Finally, breathe in, and tense from the feet upward to the chest, arms, and hands, and now tense the face, head, and brain. Feel even the sensory organs tight and tense. Every organ and every cell of your body should now be as tense as you can get it. Hold the tension for a moment, and then as you release your breath, first let go of the tension in the head and face, down through the neck, the shoulders, the arms and hands, down all the way to the feet. Let all the tension melt away.

As you inhale, repeat this last full–body tensing once more, all the way up into your face and brain, feeling every cell in your body tensed, and now, as you exhale, release from the top down, until every part of your body is relaxed.

Now, as you lie relaxed, take a gentle breath in, and as you release that breath, feel yourself melting into the floor, with no tension anywhere in your body. Breathe normally, and just lie there for a few minutes, feeling completely relaxed.

As you do this exercise, notice any parts of your body where it seems harder to release the tension. Learning to recognize tension in your body is the first step toward learning to let it go.

YOGA SELF–MASSAGE

Yoga and massage are similar in many ways. Both activate areas along the spine, help to wake up joints, and improve the circulation of both blood and lymph. The following series of yoga postures provides an "internal massage" for the spine, joints, and internal organs. Use it as a warm-up before your exercise. You may want to read the following instructions into your tape recorder and play it back whenever you wish to perform the movements.

SPINAL STRETCH   Lie on the floor with your arms relaxed at your sides. Breathing in through the nose, slowly raise your arms over your head so that they are stretched out on the floor behind you. At the same time that you are

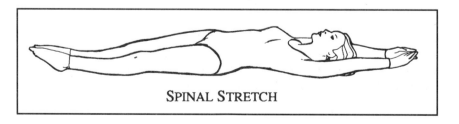

SPINAL STRETCH

inhaling and bringing your arms back, point your toes so that you are stretching from the waist down to your toes and from your waist up to your fingertips. Hold in your breath and feel the tension of the stretch in your spine and in the entire length of your body. Release the tension without changing position, and relax around the held breath for a moment. Then exhale, bringing your arms back to your sides. Lie flat, breathing normally, and relax, enjoying the benefits of the stretch. This lying position, known as the Resting Pose, is one of the most important postures in yoga. Take the time to experience the total relaxation that the name implies. Repeat the spinal stretch three times.

KNEES TO CHEST Lying on your back, bring both knees to the chest, with the arms clasped around your knees, holding one wrist with the other hand. Relax in this folded-up position, breathing in and out normally. Feel the invigorating stretch in your lower back. Now, still holding this position, rock gently from side to side to wake up the spine. Release your knees and straighten the legs, lowering them slowly to the floor, returning to the Resting Pose. Rest for a while and enjoy the feeling relaxation. Repeat three times.

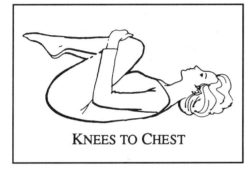

KNEES TO CHEST

COBRA Roll over onto your tummy. Lie flat with your toes together, your forehead on the floor, and your palms flat on the floor next to the armpits. Breathe in, slowly raising the head and neck. Open your eyes and look up through the eyebrows. Continuing to breathe in, rise further, lifting the chest off the floor and curling the spine back as far as possible without lifting the hips or pelvis off the floor. Hold your breath in this reverse stretch, looking up through the eyebrows and jutting the chin out with the teeth together, tensing the throat and neck. Hold this position for several seconds, then begin to exhale. Lower the stomach to the floor, then the chest, and finally allow the head to roll forward to the floor. Relax in a lying position on your tummy with your head to one side. Repeat this posture three times.

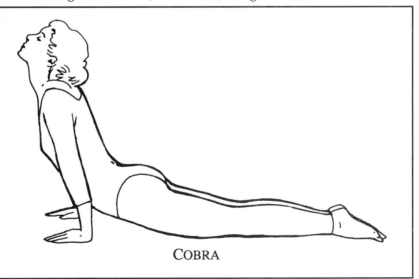

COBRA

CANINE STRETCH   Still lying on your tummy on the floor, place your palms next to your armpits and push yourself up, with your weight on your hands and the balls of your feet. Straighten your legs and raise your buttocks

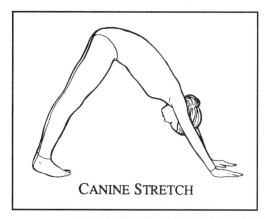

CANINE STRETCH

in the air, as if a rope were lifting your lower spine toward the ceiling. Hold this position for a few moments. Really push up your lower back area, feeling the spinal stretch. Then bend your knees, lower your body to the floor position, and relax. Breathe in and out normally throughout this exercise; do not hold your breath. For a different stretch and a different sensation, try drawing your heels down to the floor in the raised position, rather than keeping your weight on your toes. Repeat the Canine Stretch three times, ending in the floor position.

PRENATAL POSTURE   From lying on the floor, push yourself up into a kneeling position, so that you are sitting relaxed on your feet, with the tops of the feet flat on the floor, the toes touching, and the heels turned out to the sides. Take a deep, slow inhalation. Extend your arms out in front of you with the fingers lightly touching, exhale slowly, and as you exhale,

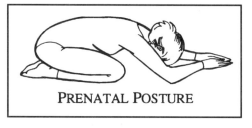

PRENATAL POSTURE

bend forward until your forehead is resting on the floor with your arms extended. Relax in this position, breathing normally, for at least one minute. Repeat three times. This position, known as the Prenatal Posture, stimulates the circulation of blood to the head, making your mind alert and your eyes rested and bright.

DIGESTION TONING POSTURES

Performing these Digestion Toning Postures will help to relax your entire digestive and eliminative systems. They are great to do any time, but especially if you feel abdominal discomfort. These exercises are done in the head–down, antigravity position on the slant board, bringing blood into the abdominal organs to nourish their tissues and carry away nutrients for the rest of the body. The movements are based on yoga postures designed to stimulate and tone the muscles and nerve centers that control digestion. By helping to overcome sluggishness of the stomach, intestines, and liver, these postures encourage proper elimination and speed the purification process.

ABDOMINAL CONTRACTION   Lying on your back on the slant board, exhale all the breath from your lungs, and once again draw in your abdominal muscles, making your waist as small as you can. Keeping your lungs deflated, draw your chest toward your chin, tensing the abdominal muscles at the same time. Pull everything in and up inside. Then relax and breathe normally. Repeat the exercise ten times, then relax in the resting pose.

LEG RAISES   Still lying on the slant board, raise both legs together. Keep the legs straight and the toes pointed. Raise your legs slowly until they are vertical with respect to the room, then lower them as slowly as possible, keeping your attention on the slow, smooth movement. Notice the toning pull in your abdominal muscles. Repeat the leg raises ten times.

BICYCLING   Lying on the slant board, pedal your legs in the air, holding the legs vertical and allowing your thighs to push forcefully against the abdominal organs with each cycling motion. Pedal briskly, about two cycles per second. Keep pedaling for one to three minutes, depending on your level of fitness, feeling the beneficial toning in the abdominal organs.

PLOUGH POSTURE   Lying on the slant board, raise your legs up and all the way back behind your head, as far back as you can comfortably go. Keep your knees straight and feel the pull. If you are very limber, you may be able to go all the way back and touch the board behind your head. Keep your arms at your sides, but if you need a little extra support, you may prop up your buttocks with your hands, resting on bent elbows. Once you have your feet all the way back, breathe normally and hold the pose as long as it is comfortable. For an extra stretch in the lower back, try bringing your arms back behind your head. While in the plough position, you may also try to lower your knees down toward the slant board, next to your ears, to provide a different stretch. Do not force your movements; just do what is comfortable for you. With a little practice, this posture will become much easier. Slowly lower your legs back onto the slant board and relax in the resting pose, feeling the effects of this rejuvenating yoga stretch.

PALMING   Lying on the slant board, rub your palms together until you feel the heat, cup your hands over your closed eyes, and feel the relaxation spreading to the muscles of your face and all through your body. Continue palming until the heat is gone from your hands.

YOGA REJUVENATION POSTURES

The ancient system of hatha yoga had a profound understanding of the importance of glandular health, and many yoga postures are designed to stimulate and balance the function of the various endocrine glands. On Day 20, your evening activity will include these rejuvenation postures, which have been used for centuries to preserve youth and extend life expectancy. Practice these postures regularly to keep your glands young and healthy. If you wish, read the instructions into your tape recorder so that you can perform these postures in smooth, flowing movements without interruptions.

KNEES TO CHEST   Lie on the floor in the resting pose, with your arms at your sides. Relax and breathe for a few minutes. Now, bring both knees to the chest with your arms clasped around your knees. Relax in this position, breathing in and out normally and feeling the stretch in the lower back. Hold this position and rock gently from side to side for a minute or so. Stop rocking, and with your knees still to your chest, relax again for another minute or two, then release and straighten your knees, lower your legs slowly to the floor, and rest for a few minutes in the resting pose. This knee–to–chest posture is excellent for relaxing the lower back and easing back strain.

ROCKING PLOUGH   Raise your legs with the knees straight and grab your ankles, or as far down your legs as you can comfortably reach. Now, slowly pull your legs down toward your trunk, tuck your head forward, and gently rock forward and back on your spine. Rock as far back as you can comfortably go, if you are very flexible, you may be able to touch the floor behind your head with your toes. Do not strain. Now, let go of your ankles, and if you can, bring your legs all the way back behind your head with the knees straight, supporting your lower back with your hands resting on your elbows, and relax in this inverted position. While your legs are back there, bend your knees and bring them down toward the ears and relax in this position. Then straighten your knees again, return to the Rocking Plough position, begin to rock gently, and rock forward and sit up.

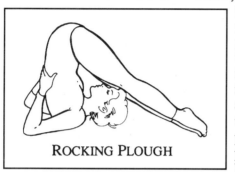

ROCKING PLOUGH

SEATED TOE PULL   Sit quietly for a moment, then as you breathe out bend forward and grab your big toes and pull on them. According to many yoga teachers, this toe–pull stimulates the pituitary gland. Release your toes and sit up. Now, as you inhale, raise your arms above your head. As you breathe out, bend forward, with your arms reaching as far down your leg as they will go and your head as close to your knees as possible. Keep your knees straight and breathe normally. Relax in this position for as long as you can, then breathe in and sit up. Breathe out and bend forward with your head toward your knees again, and relax as long as you can in the down position, breathing normally.

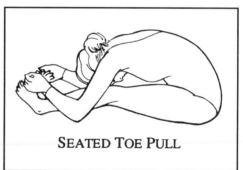

SEATED TOE PULL

HIGH SHOULDER STAND   Lie down again and relax in the resting pose. Now, bring your legs up with your knees straight and push off with your arms, supporting your lower back with your hands resting on bent elbows. Push your body up until you are in a completely vertical inverted position, with your weight on the top of the spine and the back of the neck. This is one of the most invigorating and rejuvenating yoga postures, because it reverses the effects of gravity. Support your lower back with your hands and breathe normally into your abdomen. Bend your chin into your neck to stimulate the thyroid gland. With your legs straight up in the air, rotate your ankles, first in one direction, then the other. If you are still comfortable in this position, spread your legs far out to the sides and rotate your ankles. Bring your legs back together, still breathing normally, and do a forward and back split with your legs, with first one leg forward, then the other. Come out

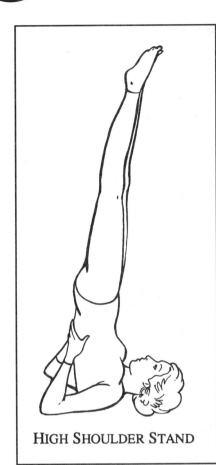

HIGH SHOULDER STAND

of this inverted posture the same way you got into it, letting your legs drop back behind your head, bracing your hands on the floor, and gradually rolling back down on the spine. Pay close attention as you roll back, trying to release one vertebra at a time. Relax in the resting pose, feeling the effects of the posture.

FISH POSE. The Fish Pose is a perfect complement to the shoulder stand. Lie on your back and breathe normally. Begin by doing the "easy fish." Put your weight on your elbows and arch your back, letting your head drop back so that your weight is resting partially on your elbows and partially on the very top of your head. Your back should form an arch from the buttocks to the top of your head. Let your hands rest on your hip joints. This is a wonderful position for stimulating the thyroid, the thymus, and the glands in the head. Now, slide back down into the resting position and relax, enjoying the benefits.

FULL FISH POSE. Cross your legs at the ankles with the knees bent and pull on both big toes. Pull your toes down behind the opposite knees. Now, keeping your hands on your toes, try to drop your knees down to the floor. Feel the stretch and pull on the hip joints and thigh muscles. In this position, go into the Fish Pose once more. Push up with your weight on your elbows and the top of your head. Then slide your head and arms back down, slide your legs forward and relax, feeling the invigorating effects of this posture.

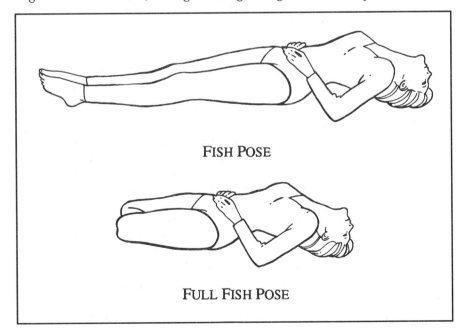

FISH POSE

FULL FISH POSE

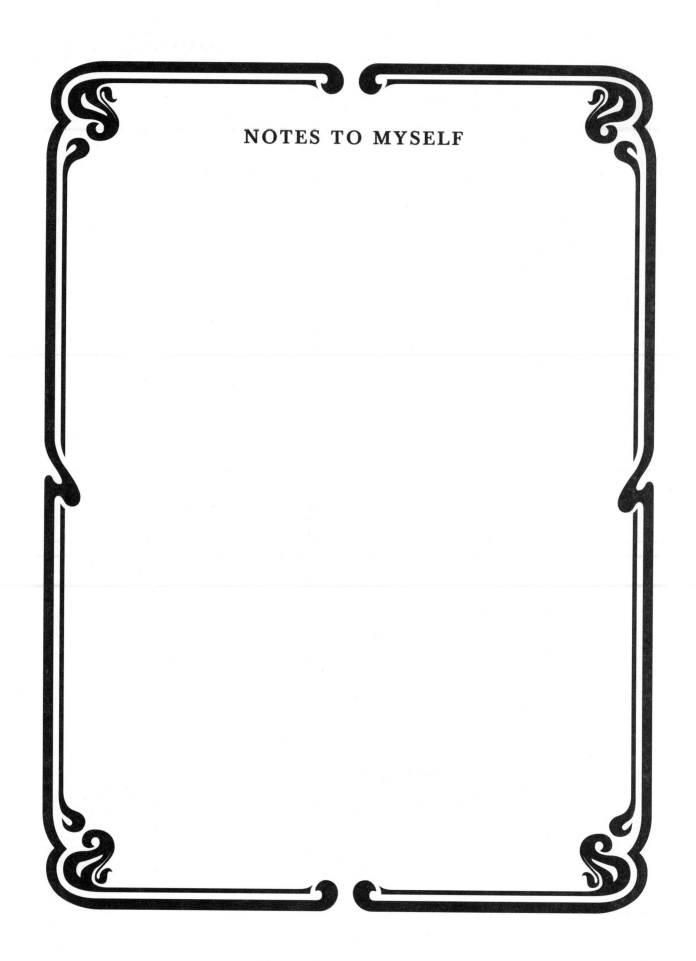

NOTES TO MYSELF

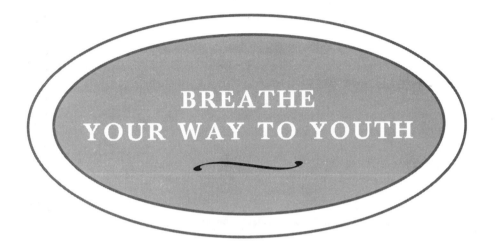

BREATHE YOUR WAY TO YOUTH

*B*reathing is the only bodily function that can be both consciously controlled and automatic. Our intelligent marine friends, the whales and dolphins, must take every breath consciously, and, therefore, can sleep for only a few moments at a time. We humans, however, allow the muscles that control breathing to breathe for us as we go about our business, letting our bodies automatically adjust our intake of air, depending on our level of activity or our emotions.

Beyond automatic breathing, we also have the opportunity to regulate our own breath, and, by so doing, to establish a connection between our conscious and unconscious functions. We can use our breath to change our energy level or our mood. In fact, taking control of your breath is a very important step toward taking control of your health and self–awareness.

I am going to show you how to establish a new, conscious breathing habit that is basic to my Cleansing and Rejuvenation Program. When practiced daily, youthful breathing will give you a glowing appearance, greater vitality, and increased alertness.

REJUVENATION THROUGH BREATH

Because the aging process takes place within the individual cells of the body, staying youthful depends on maintaining cellular health. Two critical factors in preventing aging are the oxygenation and detoxification of the cells. Proper breathing is essential to both these functions.

Oxygen is our most vital nutrient. We can live without food for weeks and

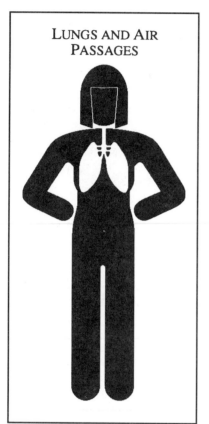

LUNGS AND AIR
PASSAGES

without water for days, but without air we can live only a few minutes. Oxygen nourishes the cells and burns the waste that would otherwise accumulate in them. The more oxygen we deliver to the cells, the more our tissues can be cleansed and rejuvenated with each breath.

Your lungs are like two bunches of grapes, except that the grapes are microscopic air chambers called alveoli. Tiny blood capillaries surround the walls of these alveolar air spaces like a fine net. The oxygen in the air you breathe is transferred across the thin walls of the alveoli into the blood, which turns bright red as the blood picks up oxygen. The blood then returns to the heart, which pumps it via the arteries to the body's cells. The oxygen passes into the cells, where it combines with sugar or fat to give off the heat energy that powers our life processes. The by–products of this oxidation are carbon dioxide and water. The carbon dioxide passes out of the cells into the blood, which is now dark and bluish, to be carried back to the lungs. Here the carbon dioxide passes out of the alveoli into the air, and is breathed out along with some of the water. The remaining water is carried away to be eliminated by the kidneys.

Within the red blood cells are molecules of hemoglobin, an iron–containing protein that is able to pick up life–giving oxygen, carry it to the cells, and then release it. Therefore, the body's supply of oxygen depends on an adequate supply of iron in your diet. A diet full of iron–rich vegetables, such as those in the High–Iron Salad on page 106, help to maintain your hemoglobin, ensuring an adequate supply of oxygen to the cells and imparting a rosy glow to your complexion.

Many other powerful nutrients, such as those in your Oxygenation Cocktail on page 82, help to deliver oxygen to all the cells of the body. That is why I recommend adding that drink to your daily regimen!

The elimination of waste through the breath is as important as the intake of oxygen. Classical Chinese medical theory recognized this cleansing function of the lungs thousands of years ago when it classified the lungs, the skin, and the colon as a single organ system. All these organs of elimination remove toxins from the body. In fact, your skin actually breathes, too. It performs about one seventh of the body's total respiration, absorbing oxygen and eliminating carbon dioxide along with other impurities.

Give your skin a chance to breathe by wearing clothes made of natural fabrics. Wear loose clothing at home so that the air can circulate around your body. Whenever possible, take "air baths," wearing nothing at all, so that your skin can really do its job. The Friction Air Bath on page 146 is a pleasant addition to any bath or shower. Whenever the weather permits, include this invigorating skin treatment in your schedule.

If you are a smoker, or have been in the past, you will be encouraged to know that proper breathing of fresh, clean air will help to restore your lungs to their best possible condition. If one of the goals you have set for yourself is to quit smoking or cut down, correct breathing can be a powerful tool to help you carry out your resolution.

I was a smoker myself at one time. When I finally decided to quit, whenever I wanted a cigarette I would take a deep breath, which helped me relax. When I paused to take a breath, I would also notice that the desire for a cigarette was really prompted by some emotion that I was suppressing. Breathing helped me become aware of these underlying emotions so that I could deal with them. To combat the urge to smoke, I would also take a walk by the ocean where I would do deep breathing for about a half hour. The negative ions at the seashore and the salt air helped me overcome my craving for tobacco.

Of course, cigarette smoke is not the only pollutant that injures your lungs and ages your appearance. Our environment is filled with smog and other toxic substances that produce free radicals that damage all the cells of the body! To enjoy the full anti–aging benefits of youthful breathing, make use of your daily brisk walks to fill your lungs with plenty of clean air. Whenever you can, visit the seashore or the countryside to revitalize your lungs, rejuvenate your cells, and lift your spirits.

Even if you have decided to remain a smoker, or if you have bronchial asthma or sinus problems, you can still clear your lungs of congestion by using a cleansing inhalant based on essential oils. On page 156 I describe the use of essential oils to cleanse and beautify your skin, and to influence your mood, by relaxing in fragrant herbal steams and baths. Such external treatments are one form of "aromatherapy", or the use of natural aromatic plant essences. Essential oils can also be used internally, by inhaling their fumes, for their healing properties. Do not be deceived by the lovely fragrances of these plant essences. They can have potent medicinal properties, and must be treated with caution when used in inhalants.

A prepared herbal inhalant that is my personal favorite is Inspirol, a product based on the formulas of Edgar Cayce, the renowned twentieth–century psychic who formulated natural remedies for all kinds of physical dysfunctioning. This product has assisted many people in quitting smoking. Instead of inhaling a cigarette, they inhale a dose of Inspirol! It is quite stimulating energetically and as an expectorant. You can buy Inspirol in a health–food store or order it through the Source Guide in this book.

Balloon Breathing

After using the Cleansing Inhalant, you will benefit from Balloon Breathing. Balloon Breathing increases your ability to cleanse your lungs, your blood, and your cells. It is an enjoyable anti–aging practice that you can use at home, or during a break at work. Balloon breathing is used by respiratory therapists to strengthen the lungs of patients with asthma and emphysema. It is also an excellent facial exercise for keeping cheeks firm, eliminating telltale squirrel pouches, and keeping the muscles around the lips elastic.

Perform Balloon Breathing with a large, thick balloon that requires strenuous blowing. Breathe in through your nose to fill your lungs, then blow the air into the balloon, continuing until it is filled. Let the air out of the balloon and then repeat the exercise for a total of five to fifteen minutes, maintaining an awareness of your facial muscles. Balloon Breathing is a featured activity several times during your Cleansing and Rejuvenation Program.

TIPS FOR CUTTING DOWN ON SMOKING

Smokers can benefit from many elements of the 21–Day Program in their efforts to reduce their tobacco consumption. Exercise is not only healthful in itself, it also helps smokers to cut down. Research has shown that a brief period of brisk walking actually reduces the craving for the next cigarette.

A good herbal alternative to tobacco is to get a bag of licorice root, available in health–food stores, and chew or suck on a piece of root whenever you feel the urge to smoke. Many of my clients have been able to quit smoking this way. Licorice is very high in natural sugar and helps to even out irregularities in blood–sugar levels produced by smoking. It is also a mild stimulant.

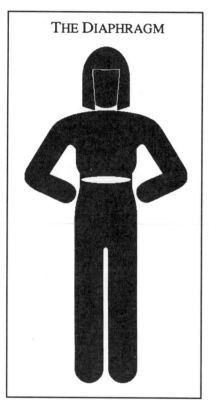

THE DIAPHRAGM

Balloon Breathing helps to clean the waste out of the lungs. People with respiratory diseases are taught to exhale through pursed lips for this same reason. Breathing against resistance helps to maintain a higher pressure in the airways, keeping them open longer so that more waste can get out, while allowing more oxygen to enter the lungs. This is why I recommend that when you do any breathing exercises you always exhale through pursed lips, as if you were whistling. In fact, whistling is another good way to clear out the breathing passages.

CONSCIOUS BREATH CONTROL

Your lungs are marvelously designed for taking in nourishing oxygen and eliminating waste, but they are completely passive in their function. They cannot expand and contract without the help of the muscles that surround them. About 80 percent of the work of breathing is done by the diaphragm, a dome-shaped sheet of muscle that divides the rib cage horizontally at about the bottom of the breastbone. It provides the floor on which the lungs and heart sit, and forms an arched dome over the liver and stomach. When the diaphragm contracts, the vertex of its bell shape flattens downward, creating a partial vacuum in the chest cavity to expand the lungs. At the same time, it presses down on the liver, stomach, and intestines, causing the belly to swell and giving the abdominal organs a stimulating massage. When you are resting or sleeping, the diaphragm alone controls breathing, but when you are tense or exercising vigorously, breathing is aided by the muscles between the ribs and in the shoulder girdle.

Breathing a full breath requires pulling the diaphragm as far down as possible to inflate the lungs completely. To exhale fully, you must push your diaphragm up. The more stale air you squeeze out of the lungs, the more toxins you remove from your body, and the more oxygen you can take in during your next refreshing, rejuvenating inhalation.

It requires conscious attention to overcome a habit of shallow breathing. Wearing tight waistbands or constricting undergarments discourages the use of anything but the upper part of the lungs. Proper breathing also requires correct posture. The straighter your spine, the more open your lungs, and the more your internal organs will be held in proper alignment.

Exercise helps to keep the diaphragm muscle toned and to increase the circulatory system's ability to carry oxygen efficiently to all the cells of the body. Vigorous activity and strong breathing help to prevent the deposit of fatty sediment on the linings of the arteries. Swimming is an excellent form of exercise for increasing your awareness of and capacity for proper breathing. If you have access to a pool, you may want to choose swimming as your exercise for today. As you do your exercise, work on developing good breathing habits, supported by proper body alignment. Use your awareness to follow your breath throughout your body.

In yoga, conscious breath control has been developed to a high level of refinement. For more than two thousand years, hatha yoga practitioners have been combining their repertoire of bodily movements with awareness of breath—the breath is equated with prana, the life force.

Breathing exercises derived from hatha yoga will help to bring your awareness and your breath into every part of your body. If you have been a shallow breather all your life, or if you haven't done breathing exercises before, you may find yourself getting a little dizzy. Take it easy; do not over-do it to begin with. These exercises cleanse and purify your whole system, while eliminating toxins and waste through the breath and bringing oxygen to all the cells.

By learning to control breath through these yogic exercises, you can achieve balance throughout your being and direct your consciousness to whatever part of your body needs cleansing, nourishing, and healing. As you continue to practice breathing exercises daily, you will begin to notice an improvement in your concentration. Your mind will become clearer and easier to focus. Apply the combination of breathing, relaxation, and concentration to any problem area in your life—it will bring you great insight and enhanced creativity.

Three–Part Breathing

Three–Part Breathing will help you to become aware of the three segments of the lungs. Most shallow breathers bring air only into the upper lungs. By breathing into the chest, the diaphragm, and the abdomen, you fill your lungs all the way to the bottom of their lower lobes. If you wish, read the instructions into your tape recorder so that you can do the activity while relaxing.

Lie flat on your back on the floor. Relax and observe your breathing pattern for a while to become familiar with your natural breathing pattern. Now, place your hands flat on the upper chest and inhale deeply through your nostrils, filling the chest. This is the only part of the breathing apparatus that the average shallow breather uses. Expand your lungs, opening the chest. Feel it expanding not only from back to front as your hands rise with the chest wall, but also out to the sides and into the back. Bring the breath all the way out to the shoulders and all through your chest.

Now, breathe out through pursed lips, feeling the chest deflate. Inhale and exhale very slowly, being fully aware of the way your breath fills and empties your chest. Repeat this process three times.

Now, place the palms of your hands over the diaphragm, just below the rib cage. Your diaphragm lies in the region just below the breasts down to the navel. Now, try to breathe just in the diaphragm area. Breathe in through your nose, but this time don't let the chest expand. Isolate the diaphragm and fill it with breath. As you inhale, feel the lower rib cage expanding, not only to the front but to the sides and back as well.

Diaphragmatic breathing has a positive effect on the emotional center in the solar plexus, bringing a sense of tranquility. Hold your breath comfortably, and then exhale slowly through pursed lips, feeling the diaphragm region deflate. Repeat three times. Don't be discouraged if you cannot do this diaphragmatic breathing right away; you are learning to move a new part of your body. As you practice this exercise during the 21–Day Program, you will improve your ability to isolate and breathe into your diaphragm.

Finally, place your hands over the lower abdomen and inhale just into that section. Do not let your chest or diaphragm expand. Breathe in through your nostrils, and feel the abdominal region expand as you inhale. Keep the expansion as you hold in the breath for a moment, then exhale through pursed lips, slowly and completely, feeling the abdomen deflate. Repeat the abdominal breathing three times.

At the end of this exercise, lie quietly for a few minutes in the resting position, breathing naturally.

Complete Breath

Now that you have practiced breathing separately in each segment of the lungs, you are ready to coordinate these three phases of breathing into one smooth, continuous, flowing breath. The Complete Breath makes optimal use of your breathing apparatus, allowing the greatest possible intake of oxygen and elimination of carbon dioxide.

Still lying on the floor, breathe in through the nostrils, filling the abdomen first, feeling it expand. Then, on the same inhalation, move the breath up to include the diaphragm and solar plexus. Still inhaling, move the breath into the chest. Now, you are completely filled with breath. Hold your breath and relax for a moment around the held breath. Feel the relaxation spread through your whole body. Now, begin to release the breath through pursed lips. Release from the top all the way down; first release the breath from the chest, then the diaphragm, and finally the abdomen. Feel the parts of your body deflate as you breathe out.

Relax and breathe normally, taking a nice deep breath. Notice the feelings in the different parts of your body. You may feel your head becoming clearer as the "cobwebs" are gently wafted away by the Complete Breath.

Now, repeat the Complete Breath. Inhale again through the nostrils, filling the abdomen, then the diaphragm, and finally the chest, in a continuous wavelike motion. As it becomes more natural for you, you may want to count. Take in your breath slowly in this wavelike, three–part motion to a count of eight–abdomen, diaphragm, and chest. Hold for four, relaxing around the held breath. Then exhale slowly for eight counts, first from the chest, then from the diaphragm, and finally the abdomen.

After just a few of these breaths, you will feel wonderfully relaxed. As you practice, breathe in positive thoughts–peace, harmony, well–being, or whatever words have special meaning for you. As you breathe in, feel the great ocean of life–energy flowing into you–abdomen, diaphragm, and chest. As you hold your breath, send this energy to every cell in your body. As you exhale, let go of all the toxins, the worries, and the negative thoughts. Continue this breathing pattern for two to five minutes. The longer you do it, the greater the benefits.

Relaxing in the resting position, allow yourself to breathe normally for a few minutes, and feel the healing, calming effects of the Complete Breath on your body, mind, and emotions. The more you practice the Complete Breath and make it a part of your life, the greater the rejuvenating effect upon your cells.

Alternate–Hemisphere Breathing

Alternate–Hemisphere Breathing, derived from hatha yoga, helps balance all the processes of the body, and promotes balanced functioning of the brain.

Sit comfortably with the spine straight. Use a straight–backed chair; or if you sit on the floor, you may put your back against a wall. Rest the right thumb lightly against the right nostril, and the ring and little finger against the left nostril. Before you begin, exhale slowly through both nostrils.

Now, hold the right nostril closed with your right thumb. Slowly and deeply inhale through the left nostril to a count of five. Keeping the right nostril closed, press the left one closed, and hold the air in your lungs for five counts. Now, open the right nostril only and exhale to a count of five.

Without pausing, inhale through the right nostril to a count of five, press the right nostril closed, and hold for five counts. Now, open the left nostril and exhale through it for five counts.

Repeat this cycle ten times to begin with, gradually increasing to twenty as you continue your daily practice. Do not slow down or speed up your breathing, but keep it going at the same slow, regular pace.

Only recently, Western research has shown that this ancient breathing technique is a powerful way to control brain function. Scientists at the Salk Institute and the University of California at San Diego have found that we breathe primarily through one nostril for one to three hours, and then switch to the other. When the left nostril is active, the right–brain hemisphere dominates our thinking, and when the right nostril is dominant, the left hemisphere is more active.

Check and see which of your nostrils is clearest at any time during the day. When the right nostril is clear, that is a good time for left–brain activity, such as logical thinking or working with numbers. When your left nostril is clear, that is a good time to do right–brain activities involving intuition, spatial relations, and creative and artistic endeavors.

By taking voluntary control of your breathing, you can actually influence your brain activity. If you breathe through the congested nostril, you can switch brain dominance to the opposite hemisphere. So, if you need to do something creative, breathe through the left nostril to stimulate right–brain activity. If you need to balance your checkbook, breathe through your right nostril for a few minutes to stimulate the left brain. You can use Inspirol, the cleansing inhalant I described on page 135, to help clear the air passages and facilitate the switch from one nostril to the other.

Alternate Breathing is also restful when you have difficulty falling asleep. Try it tonight after your bath, before you retire.

BREATHING AWAY STRESS

Breathing is one of your most valuable methods for releasing tension, anxiety, and stress. When you learn to breathe deeply, you begin to release emotional tension that has been trapped in the abdominal area. The solar plexus, a network of nerve fibers in the abdomen, is the emotional center of the physical body. From the solar plexus, nerve impulses control all the abdominal organs and regulate nutrition, assimilation, and growth. Improper, shallow breathing can cause the buildup of nervous tension, because it cuts us off from the feelings centered in the abdomen.

Many of my clients suffer from constipation or sexual problems. We often find that a large part of their difficulty is that they are not breathing in their abdomen. As they direct attention and breath into the abdominal organs, they suddenly bring life to this part of the body.

One client, Melinda, never had orgasms until she learned to breathe correctly. Distraught over a relationship, she had followed a friend's advice and begun attending yoga classes. One day in class, she was sitting on the floor in a yoga posture, with one leg bent in toward the groin and the other leg extended out to the side. As instructed, she leaned over the extended leg, reached out to grasp the ankle, and began to breathe deeply into the pelvis. "You may never have thought of breathing this way," the teacher commented, "but open up the pelvic area with your breath." Suddenly, Melinda began to feel sexual excitement. How could this be happening to her, in this room full of earnest spiritual students? From the moment on, working with her breath, she underwent a sexual awakening. Eventually, she was able to use her breath to encourage full sexual feelings.

Many people unconsciously hold their breath during sex. Are you one of them? With practice, you can learn to use your breath to bring full awareness into your sexual organs. Many sex therapists and body workers are specially trained to work with the breath to help clients achieve sexual satisfaction. Natural birthing techniques also recognize the importance of breath.

Just as breathing helps to expel waste from your body, it is also a powerful way to eliminate negative thoughts. Use your breathing to inhale peace, harmony, and well–being, and to release all your worries and tensions. Whenever you feel anxious or tense, stop for a few moments, take a deep inhalation, breathing in the oxygen, the life–energy, and the positive thoughts that nourish your system, and breath out, long and slow, to release the tension and anxiety from every part of your body.

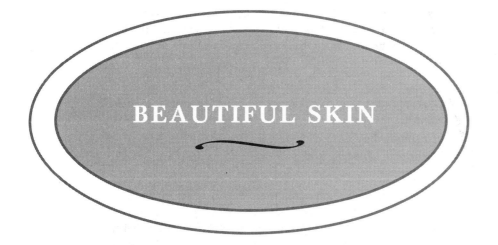

BEAUTIFUL SKIN

*B*EAUTIFUL *S*KIN: *F*ROM THE *I*NSIDE OUT

Your skin is the mirror of your health. When you are well nourished, adequately exercised, and free of toxins and wastes, your skin will be smooth, unblemished, and youthful looking–it will glow with an inner radiance. Your hair and nails, which are an extension of the skin, will be strong and healthy as well.

Did you know that the skin is your body's largest organ? Wrapped around you at a thickness of only one–twentieth of an inch, your skin weighs about six pounds. This thin layer of tissue performs several very important functions. It serves as a protective covering, keeping your body fluids in and harmful materials out. The skin regulates body temperature through a network of blood vessels just below the surface, which expand or contract to control how much blood is brought to the surface to be cooled by evaporating sweat. Your sense of touch–pain, pressure, light touch, warmth, and cold–depends on specialized nerve endings in the epidermis near the skin surface.

An often overlooked function of the skin is its vital role as an organ of elimination. About one third of the body's impurities are excreted through the skin—more than one pound of wastes each day! Your sweat glands not only regulate body temperature, but they also function like miniature kidneys that cleanse the system of impurities. In fact, sweat has almost the same chemical makeup as urine, and if the pores are choked with dead cells, uric acid and other wastes will remain in the body, forcing the other organs of elimination to work harder. Many of these toxins and wastes end up lodged in the skin tissues, producing a mottled or sallow appearance.

The traditional Chinese medical system recognizes the relationship between the skin and other organs. By looking at the skin on certain areas of the body, Chinese doctors are able to determine the functional performance of the inner organs. This makes sense when you consider that improperly functioning internal organs will cause additional toxins to appear in the skin.

Your skin is constantly renewing itself. It actually consists of four layers. At the bottom is the basal, or growing layer, where basal cells divide to produce new cells. These new cells displace the older ones, pushing them upward through a clear cell layer and a granular layer, until they finally reach the outer, keratin layer. It takes about three to four weeks for the cells beginning at the basal layer to end up on the surface. As the cells mature, they produce granular material that eventually causes the cells to consolidate into a thick, tough outer keratin layer. Finally, the cells in this protective outer layer slough off, carrying away large molecules of waste material with them.

We sometimes forget that the skin not only moves wastes from the inside out, but is also capable of absorbing substances directly into the body. This fact was brought dramatically home to me when I observed the effects of progesterone cream that one of the doctors I work with was giving to his patients for premenstrual stress, or PMS. Applying just a little of this hormone cream to the skin often produced a remarkable improvement in the emotional ups and downs and other symptoms that are so common a few days before your period.

This absorptive power of the skin is now being employed as a way of administering medicines. Special skin patches, called derms, deliver estrogen for menopausal problems, scopolamine for motion sickness, and nitroglycerin for cardiovascular pain. Quite popular also are patches for nicotine withdrawal. Scientists are experimenting with derms for controlling diabetes, weight loss and fertility.

If beneficial substances can be so readily administered through the skin, then harmful substances can also enter our bodies in the same way. When you put on perfume, cosmetics, deodorants, or insect repellents, remember that it is not just the surface of the skin that you are affecting. The British medical journal Lancet recently reported toxic physical and mental symptoms, especially in children, from the application of insect repellent on the skin. Try to use skin–care products that contain pure and natural, recognizable ingredients.

Throughout this book I am providing you with many activities which focus on cleansing and beautifying your skin from within and without by promoting its eliminative functions. I will help you to clear it of the toxins and waste materials that produce blemishes, dry patches, furrows and wrinkles, fatty cellulite deposits, and unhealthy coloration.

BEAUTY BEYOND SKIN DEEP

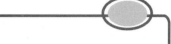

Now that you understand how your skin cells reproduce you can see how quickly you can improve your complexion. In fact, at the end of the 21–Day Program, most of your facial skin will be new. The quality of your skin depends on the quality of the raw materials from which the skin cells are made. This means that your complexion is a direct reflection of the quality of your diet.

The best diet for your skin is the Clean and Clear Diet, emphasizing fluid–rich fresh fruits and vegetables with nutrients that maintain your body's ideal acid–alkaline balance, so important to a glowing complexion. Eating right eliminates harmful saturated fats and ensures an adequate supply of GLA and EPA oils that nourish the skin and protect the heart. A healthy, youthful skin requires large doses of the vitamins and minerals in the supplement program that I recommend on page 72.

Vitamin A is essential for forming healthy cells in the basal layer and helps to enhance the skin's moisture level. A vitamin–D supplement nourishes dry skin, especially during the winter months, when it is not as readily manufactured by the body in response to exposure to sunlight. Vitamin C is an age retardant to prevent the oxidative processes that produce wrinkling of the skin and hardening of the collagen in connective tissue. Minerals that promote skin health include calcium, magnesium, zinc, manganese, and potassium.

Skin–nourishing vitamins and minerals are often helpful when applied topically as well. Vitamin–E cream or ointment, and vitamin–A and–D ointment, are very useful in preventing and correcting dry skin. One of the B vitamins, PABA, has been found to be the best topical protection against dangerous ultraviolet rays in sunlight, a principal cause of wrinkling. Some people, however, have an allergic reaction to PABA, so choose your sunscreen carefully.

Please remember that smoking, too, dries and ages the skin. If you are a smoker who has set quitting as one of your goals in this program, this is a good time to strengthen your resolve.

To counteract the unavoidable effects of aging on the skin, I recommend the twice–daily use of the natural moisturizer NaPCA.

You must drink at least eight glasses of purified water each day to properly nourish your skin. Some of this water will be supplied in herbal teas and beverages such as your morning Hot Lemon–Water Flush on page 80, your pre–exercise Oxygenation Cocktail on page 82, and the skin–food drink Rejuvelac on page 88. The rest should be provided by the Hydrating Drink on page 81. For the sake of your complexion, avoid caffeine beverages, limit or eliminate alcohol use, and stay away from diet sodas full of chemicals and caffeine.

Constipation is your complexion's worst enemy. When your colon is

FOREVER YOUNG

There really does exist a product from Sweden that rebuilds collagen and elastin! It is a totally natural compound which, when taken orally, has a rather miraculous effect on the quality of aging and sun–damaged skin. It contains natural protein and carbohydrate structures from a marine source–vitamins and minerals of the same compostition as the skin tissues.

The European research has been performed by dermatologists, biochemists, gerontologists and physiologists. After three months of daily ingestion of the product, skin thickness improved by 82% and skin elasticity improved by 25%. Significant improvements were also noticed regarding wrinkles, sun spots, dry skin, hair, and nails.

Check with your local health–food store, skin care practitioner or the Source Guide on page 231 for ordering information.

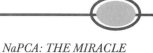

NaPCA: THE MIRACLE MOISTURIZER

NaPCA, the sodium salt of pyrrolidone carboxylic acid, is the most important natural moisturizer found in the skin. Your body manufactures NaPCA from glutamic acid, one of the amino acids that make up proteins. As skin ages, its NaPCA content decreases, so that older skin contains only half the amount found in younger skin. It is water, not oil, that keeps your skin soft and supple. NaPCA draws moisture out of the air to keep the skin hydrated and plump, helping it retain the natural resiliency of youth.

NaPCA is one of the most exciting new natural products in skin care. It is available in health–food stores in the form of a spray concentrate, often combined with aloe vera. Use it twice a day to spray your face. After bathing, you can spray your entire body. NaPCA is a wonderful moisturizer under makeup. Rather than a cosmetic cover-up, it is a natural way of correcting a deficiency that occurs with aging of the skin.

I spray my hair with NaPCA before I go to bed. In the morning, my hair looks shinier, fuller, and healthier.

clogged with waste material, your body tries to eliminate toxins through the skin. Even if your skin is functioning properly, these waste materials end up deposited in the pores and tissues. Many women, as they get older, think they need to use more makeup because their skin color has changed and their complexion has become blotchy.

Many of my clients initially decide to go on a cleansing program because they are having skin problems. Often they have tried everything, including antibiotics prescribed by a dermatologist. Not only do their skin problems not clear up satisfactorily, but many have undesirable side effects from the drugs.

Sarah is such a client of mine. She was referred to me by a skin–care specialist. When I first saw her, she had terrible acne, from her jawline all the way down to the bottom of her neck! Sarah had just lived through a stressful two years filled with some major lifestyle changes. Following her father's death, she had taken over the family business, and her own personal care had assumed very low priority. Once her business affairs were in order, she took a look at herself and realized something needed to be done. Sarah had always had some slight problems with her skin, but nothing like the massive acne that she had now.

It took us more than a year of proper diet and an internal cleansing program, in conjunction with her regular skin–care treatments, to clear her skin of acne. For Sarah, her complexion problem was a warning sign that something was the matter. The condition of her skin is her barometer to tell her when to pay more attention to her diet, her stress management, and her systems of elimination. We all have warning signs in our bodies, and for many of us, the first changes occur in the skin. When you have a sudden breakout, your body is trying to tell you that something beneath the surface needs to be corrected.

The cleansing process is not always easy. You should be aware that you may experience minor symptoms and reactions as your cleansing progresses, and the skin is one of the most common places for cleansing reactions to show up. Do not panic if you notice a new pimple or two as your stored wastes are eliminated through the skin. Your body is detoxifying and cleansing itself.

One of the most pleasurable parts of the rejuvenation program is the variety of techniques to beautify your skin through bathing, dry skin rubs, and fume baths. These procedures are easy, relaxing, and enjoyable ways to take care of yourself while indulging your senses. The results are worth it: a vibrant complexion, an energized body, and a relaxed state of mind.

DRY SKIN RUBS

Before I introduce you to the cleansing and revitalizing powers of baths and herbal steams in the next chapter, I will begin by showing how to stimulate your skin's eliminative functions with dry skin rubs.

Dry Brush Massage

Dry brush massage has many benefits. It removes the dead layers of skin and opens the pores, promotes blood circulation and lymph flow to help your body excrete toxins, stimulates the hormone–and–oil–producing glands in the skin, and invigorates the nervous system by stimulating the nerve endings. Stimulation by dry massage can help enhance immune–system function, promote muscle tone, and help break down the accumulations of fat and toxic waste known as cellulite. Regular dry brushing will accomplish these functions and also improve your overall complexion and make you look younger and feel better all over.

The only equipment you will need is a stiff bath–type brush with natural vegetable bristles. The brush should be at least the size of the palm of your hand, and should have a long handle so that you can reach all parts of your body. Avoid nylon or other synthetic bristles, because they are sharp and may damage the skin.

Begin at the soles of your feet and brush vigorously in a circular motion, moving upward gradually to massage every part of your body. Use as much pressure as you can stand, remembering that different parts of the body have different degrees of sensitivity. After brushing the feet and legs, move upward to the abdomen; then brush the hands and arms inward toward the chest. Brush down from the neck, down the back, and up from the abdomen toward the chest. Brush until your skin is rosy and glowing–about five minutes.

Remember that the brush is removing toxins and pore–clogging dead cells from the surface of your skin. Keep your brush clean by washing it periodically with soap and water and drying it in the sun or a warm place. Do not brush irritated skin, and do not brush the sensitive skin of your face.

The best time for a dry brush massage is when you wake up in the morning. Follow the massage with an invigorating shower or bath. Some people prefer a dry brush massage after bathing. During the 21–Day Program, you will be experimenting with several variations, so you can choose the one you like best.

Sea Salt Scrub

Another excellent method for stimulating the eliminative function of your skin is the Sea Salt Scrub. Use 100 percent sea salt, widely available at grocery and health–food stores. Place four of five generous handfuls of salt in a plastic container. In another container, put a little water, about a quart, as hot as you can stand. This will open your pores. Sitting or standing in a dry bathtub, take a soft sea sponge, dip it into the container of hot water, and wet down one part of your body at a time–your arm from the wrist to the elbow, for example. Then rub in the dry sea salt with your hand. If it is too abrasive, you can add a little water to the container of salt to make a paste, if you wish. Rub the salt on your skin with circular motions. Proceed to cover your whole body with the salt, from your feet up the legs; from your hands up the arms; and from your neck down toward the chest. Use a long–handled brush to rub the sea salt onto your back. Scrub with circular strokes until your body has a pink, healthy, warm glow.

Now, relax (as best you can) for about ten minutes. You will begin to feel your body tingle pleasantly. As the salt dries, it is drawing the toxins out of your skin. Rinse off in a warm shower, followed by a thirty–second cold splash. If your skin is very reactive, it may flush pink for a day or so. Avoid getting salt on the mucous membranes.

There are several ready–made Sea Salt Scrubs available in health food stores.

Friction Air Bath

Exposure to fresh air is very beneficial for the skin. It promotes all the skin's normal functions and aids the cleansing process. An air bath, combined with a dry skin rub, is wonderfully invigorating and promotes a clear, healthy complexion.

You may give yourself an air bath after any bath or shower. Before drying off as usual, when the weather permits, wrap yourself in a towel, go outside, and let yourself dry naturally in the fresh air. Even if you haven't got wet, you may simply go outdoors, completely naked, and expose your skin to the air. If you do not have access to a private place outdoors, or during bad weather, you can take your air bath indoors with the windows open.

After your air bath, warm yourself by rubbing your skin with a rough towel or doing a dry brush rub, to rid the skin of excreted waste material. You may do the dry rub inside or outdoors, depending on the weather.

Whenever you have the time, try this combination of bathing, air bath, and dry skin rub to provide a complete workout for your skin.

BEAUTY BONUS FACIALS

During a cleansing program, it is important to pay close attention to your skin, since some toxins released from your cells will be excreted through your pores. Facials help to tone and balance your skin, keeping it silky, healthy, and clean.

Egg–Yolk Mask

Separate the yolk from the white of an egg and save the white for use in the oatmeal–egg white pack listed below. Beat the yolk until it is frothy, and dab it onto your face, allowing it to dry and harden. Rinse the dried egg yolk from your face with cold water. The egg–yolk mask helps to moisturize dry skin.

Oatmeal Egg–White Pack

Mix one handful of raw oatmeal with one egg white and a few drops of fresh lemon juice to form a paste. Spread the paste on your face and throat, rubbing it into the areas around the chin and nose. As you allow this facial mask to dry, you will feel it soothing and tightening your skin. Remove it with splashes of cold water. This facial mask helps to smooth rough, bumpy skin, and tighten wrinkles and furrows.

Cucumber Cleansing Facial

Cucumber juice is a great natural treatment for the complexion. It helps to soften hardened skin, soothes sunburn, and gently bleaches dark spots and freckles. It has an astringent effect that will leave your face feeling wonderfully cleansed and refreshed.

Apply thin slices of fresh cucumber to your face. Cover the cucumber slices with a washcloth dipped in very hot water and wrung out. Let the facial stay on for fifteen minutes, then remove the cucumber slices, splash your face with cold water, and pat dry.

A cucumber facial is one of the beauty treatments that you could spend a lot of money for in a salon, but that you can easily do at home.

Yogurt Toning Mask

The Yogurt Toning Mask is a rejuvenating beauty treatment that takes only seconds to apply. You will feel its deep cleansing effect as it penetrates the pores to remove obstructing wastes. When used regularly, yogurt facials refine and smooth the texture of the skin.

Combine one–half cup of plain yogurt with a little fresh lemon juice. Apply it to your face and keep in on while you bathe, about twenty minutes. The mask will tighten and dry on your face.

The tingly, cooling sensation of the yogurt contrasts refreshingly with the heat of your bath. After you bath, remove the mask with splashes of cold water.

Hot Olive–Oil Rejuvenating Facial

Hot olive oil applied to the face, throat, and neck helps to moisturize and rejuvenate the skin and guard against wrinkles.

Warm a quarter–cup of olive oil. Smooth it over your face and neck, all the way down to the chest.

For added benefit, wrap a hot towel around your neck so that the oil can really seep into this area that often becomes prematurely wrinkled. Lie back in a relaxing, fragrant bath and enjoy the soothing richness of the olive oil as it penetrates your skin and refreshes your complexion. At the end of your bath, you may remove the olive oil with cleansing bath gel or other gentle bath soap or leave in on your skin for deeper penetration.

Milk Eye Packs

Dip cotton balls in warm or cold milk and place them over your eyes while you soak in your bath. Milk helps to cleanse and nourish the delicate skin around your eyes.

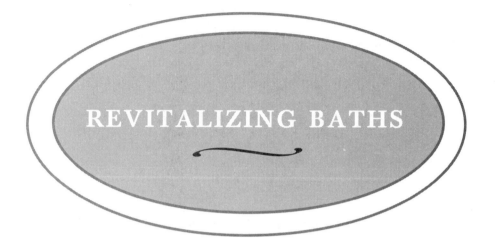

REVITALIZING BATHS

*W*hat can be more relaxing after a long, busy day than to soak in a fragrant, cleansing bath? Many people tend to cleanse themselves in a very utilitarian way–they jump in the shower, soap themselves down, rinse off, and hop out. But a bath can do so much more. It is a way to gently unwind, soothe tired muscles, open your pores, and draw wastes and toxins out through your skin. The time you take for a leisurely bath is precious personal time well invested in your health, beauty, and inner peace.

Bathing has always been a treasured ritual of personal hygiene, healing and relaxation–from the great public baths of Rome, to the elegant bath ceremonies of the Orient, the sacred healing water rituals of ancient Greece, or the fashionable European spas. Your bathroom can be a sanctuary, a private retreat from the hustle and bustle of the world outside. As you luxuriate in the fragrant aromatic essences, the healing mineral salts, and the stimulating and relaxing effects of a daily water ritual, you will come to appreciate how bathing can be a way of cleansing your body of waste and your mind of stressful thought.

Different bath temperatures have different effects on the system. Hot water is very enervating. It is a great natural tranquilizer and muscle relaxant, and many people find a hot bath just before bedtime a perfect cure for insomnia. Warm baths are very pleasant, refreshing, and relaxing. Because you can stay in warm water for a long time, it helps to maximize the cleansing and healing effects of the salts or oils that you add to your bath. Cold baths are very stimulating. You may shudder at the thought of a cold bath or shower, but as your body becomes accustomed to brief exposures to cold water, you will begin to realize its benefits.

I remember when I was a girl, my mother always told me I should end my showers with cold water. Really, it was very sound folk wisdom. A cold shower might actually be considered as close to a cure–all as any other use of water I will suggest in this book. It rejuvenates the entire system—enhancing circulation, increasing muscle tone, and activating the nervous system. It stimulates the endocrine glands, improves digestion, and speeds up metabolism, and if used regularly, it can increase resistance to infections and colds.

Throughout the program, I will be stressing hot baths for specific reasons, but I want to encourage you to use warm, cool, and even cold baths and showers just as often. The temperature of your bath will be determined partly by the time of day. A hot bath at night can be very relaxing and help you fall asleep, while a cold shower in the morning can help to wake up your entire system.

It is not wise to use hot water too often. Hot baths tend to dry out the skin because they draw the body's natural oils out of the skin. You may think that by adding oil to your bath you are putting oil into your skin, but bath oils simply rise to the surface of the water and do not add moisture to the skin. To protect your skin before taking a hot bath, oil your entire body before getting into the water. If you have dry skin, use almond oil, castor oil, olive oil, or peanut oil. If you have normal to oily skin and you take a lot of hot baths, use safflower oil, sesame oil, or sunflower oil.

I recommend that you always splash your body with cold water following a hot or warm bath or shower. After being exposed to hot water, your skin is quite sensitive to cold, because the pores are open. A cold splash invigorates the system by reducing excess body heat, closing the pores, and preventing the oils from seeping out. If you cannot bear the thought of standing under a cold shower, sponge yourself off with cold water. Over time, your body will get accustomed to the temperature change, and you will begin to relish a cold splash. Incidentally, you will also find that a cold sponging or a quick cold shower after a hot bath at night does not interfere with sleep, but helps you to relax even more.

One of the most invigorating kinds of shower is a contrast of alternating hot and cold. This stimulates all the body functions, especially the glandular system. It revitalizes skin function and improves circulation. Always be sure to finish a contrast shower with cold water. To prevent chilling afterward, wrap in a bath towel or do a dry skin rub to warm yourself.

Before a long, luxurious bath, it is a good idea to take a quick shower first, as is the Japanese custom, to get the day's grime off your body. When cleansing your skin, please avoid commercial deodorant soaps, because they are very drying. Many delightful moisturizing soaps are available in health–food stores and body–care shops, such as those made with an olive–oil or glycerin base, or with other beneficial oils. Many people use Ivory soap because it does not contain a lot of chemicals. Review the labels on soaps; remember that your skin has absorptive qualities.

While you should not expose your skin to harmful chemicals, bathing does offer an opportunity to beautify your skin and delight your senses with the aromatic essences of plants. The art and science of using natural plant essences for healing and beauty is known as aromatherapy. Although it was given that name during the present century, the use of plant essences dates back to prehistory. From the Orient to Europe and the New World, from ancient times to modern, aromatic flowers, barks, and leaves have been prized for their healing, preservative, and beautifying powers. It was not until the Middle Ages that the great Arab physician Avicenna discovered the method of distilling the pure essentials oils from plants. Herbal remedies and essential oils were an important part of medicine in the Middle Ages and the Renaissance, but gradually, with the birth of modern pharmacology, these natural substances were displaced by their more powerful synthetic forms. Now, essential oils are being rediscovered by practitioners of aromatherapy and herbal medicine as we seek gentler, lasting methods of healing and rejuvenation.

Essential oils are very readily absorbed by the skin, and inhaling their fragrance in steam also has an effect on both the mind and the body. Adding the beneficial effects of essential oils to the healing properties of water offers a very wide range of possibilities for relaxation, rejuvenation, invigoration, and beautification. I will be giving you recipes for baths and steams and other uses of essential oils throughout this chapter. You will learn how to use essential oils to revitalize and moisturize the skin, stimulate the systems of elimination, and influence your mental and emotional states. You may wish to refer to the table Curative Properties of Essential Oils on page 156 to customize the recipes to suit your own physical or emotional requirements.

Whether it is a hot soak, a fume bath, a sauna, steam room, or mud bath, the benefits of bathing are essentially the same. Bathing opens the pores and pulls the waste–laden sweat out of the system, promoting the function of your skin as an organ of elimination, and restoring its youthful, glowing color and smooth, clear texture. Minerals and herbs added to your bath amplify the healing, cleansing, and beautifying properties of water.

Besides the stimulating and relaxing effects of baths of different temperatures, water can also be used for mechanical stimulation of the skin and circulation in a manner similar to massage. You may be familiar with the wonderfully relaxing effect of a Jacuzzi. If you have a hand–held shower spray in your bathtub, you can use it to direct water at tense, painful areas on your body for a spot hydromassage. In your yard, you can use a garden hose with the water turned on full strength. For a stimulating leg massage, direct the hose at your feet, ankles, and up the legs, moving toward the center of the body. This garden hydromassage promotes circulation, tones the tissues, and helps to break down cellulite. When you are at the beach, use the powerful energy of breaking waves to massage your entire body. Stand in the water where the waves can break against painful or tense areas, or lie in the shallow water and let the surf break against you. To soothe your ankles and feet, walk along the water's edge through the foaming surf.

FUME BATHS

Steam baths, or fume baths, use intense heat to open the pores of the skin and draw the toxins out of the system. By adding various herbal preparations to the steam, you can produce specific cleansing, healing, and beautifying effects. At the Inner Beauty Institute, my clients sit in a steam cabinet with essential oils. You may want to take advantage of the steam bath in a local health club or gym, but you can also enjoy the benefits of a fume bath by making your own at home.

Aromatic Fume Bath

Prepare a steaming unit, using an electric vaporizer, a partially covered electric frying pan, or an old electric coffeepot or tea kettle. Half–fill the container with water to make the steam, plug it in (using an extension cord if necessary), and place it in an empty, dry bathtub or shower. (Be certain the tub or shower is dry to avoid electric shock). Place a chair or stool over the steaming apparatus, and sit down carefully. Drape a "tent" around you, made out of a large blanket or shower curtain. Leave an opening for your head, draping a bath towel around your neck to keep the steam in; or you may prefer to keep your head inside the tent. Sit inside the tent, which will fill rapidly with steam, for about twenty minutes. Be sure to wrap up in a towel afterward to prevent chilling.

For healing and beautifying benefits, there are a variety of herbal preparations that you can add to your fume bath. Witch hazel is wonderfully detoxifying and cleansing. Add witch hazel, widely available in pharmacies, to your steaming device before you turn it on. The witch hazel should constitute one fourth of the total liquid volume. You can also use a healing essential oil, consulting the table on page 156 to guide your selection. Some of my favorites are: lavender, excellent for relieving headaches, menstrual cramps, stress, and skin eruptions; chamomile, to relax away tension and induce sleepiness; and sandalwood, a great skin moisturizer and meditation enhancer. Add six to eight drops of essential oil on top of the water in the steaming unit

Easy Steam

For a quick fume bath that requires little preparation, try this variation as an accompaniment to a tub bath.

Put some water in an electric frying pan or vaporizer and plug it into your bathroom outlet. If you choose to use a frying pan, place it on a dry surface near the tub. Add some almond oil to the water, as well as a few drops of essential oils that you have chosen for your bath. The almond oil adds to the moisturizing benefits of the steam, imparts a delightful fragrance, and serves as a carrier for the essential oils. Prepare a hot bath, adding the aromatic oils of your choice. Keep the bathroom door closed, sit in your bath, and let the scented steam fill the room.

While you stretch out in your tub or sit in your fumebath, relax and visualize the toxins leaving your skin. Feel your sweat glands and pores opening to expel impurities. Close your eyes and picture the dead cells gently floating off the surface of your skin. Picture the minerals or herbal aromas flowing in, cleansing and nourishing your skin, making it smooth and clear.

Breathe deeply and inhale the marvelous scent that rises in the steam around you. The relaxed, pleasant mood that this fume bath produces is an important part of my program for youthful, beautiful skin. Stress can take a toll on your complexion, and relaxation can help to smooth out the frown line and wrinkles, and promote the flow of nourishing blood and oxygen into the tissues.

MAKE YOUR OWN HYDRATING BATH SALTS

Enjoy the mineralizing and cleansing benefits of Epsom salts, the moisturizing effects of castor and carrot oils, and the heady aroma and complexion–enhancing properties of the floral and fruit oils.

4 pound box of Epsom salts
4 ounces castor oil
1 teaspoon orange essential oil
1 teaspoon rose essential oil
1 teaspoon chamomile essential oil
1/2 teaspoon carrot essential oil

In a small jar, combine the castor oil with the essential oils. Pour the oil mixture over the Epsom salts. Allow the salts to stand for at least twenty-four hours so that the essences are completely absorbed. You will be using your Hydrating Bath Salts throughout the program.

You may keep the Epsom salts in the original box, but I prefer to transfer the Epsom salts to a covered glass jar, so that the cardboard box will not absorb the oils. Two handfuls (about one ounce) of the Hydrating Bath Salts added to your bath will be just right.

You may vary this recipe, adding other essential oils from the table on page 156 to produce your own personal combination of scents and healing and cleansing properties. You may also add a packet of concentrated seawater (available in powder form at aquarium stores) to the Epsom salts, to add the benefits of concentrated sea minerals to your bath. You may enjoy these bath salts throughout the year.

EPSOM SALTS SOAK

Epsom salts, or magnesium sulfate, are an age–old favorite for hot soaks. Epsom salts are available in pharmacies, supermarkets, and health–food stores. During this soak, you will be submerged in the water as deeply as possible so that your natural cooling mechanisms will not be operating. Holding the heat in the body promotes the detoxifying and drawing properties of the Epsom salts.

Pour two whole pounds of Epsom salts into a hot bath, as hot and deep as you can stand. (Cover the outflow in your bathtub if you want to raise the water to a higher level.) Soak for twenty minutes, then get out, wrap yourself in a towel or blanket, and lie down and continue to seat. You may want to cover your bed with a plastic drop cloth or other waterproof covering.

The minerals in the Epsom salts, followed by vigorous sweating, really draw the toxins out of your skin. An Epsom salts soak is wonderfully relaxing before bedtime, and is an important part of the cleansing process during the light diet that will occur on Days 14, 15, and 16.

For a luxurious, skin–soothing fragrance, you may wish to mix a few tablespoons of Hydrating Bath Salts into your soak. Since the purpose of this bath is to overheat the body, I do not recommend a cold sponging or shower afterward.

SEA–MINERAL BATH

Taking a Sea–Mineral Bath is like soaking your body in a warm tropical ocean.

Dissolve three or four pounds of sea salt in a tub of warm to hot water. The temperature of the water has a relaxing effect and helps your body absorb the valuable minerals in the sea salt. Relax and soak for twenty minutes. Remember that the fluids inside your body are in many ways chemically similar to the water of the ocean. So it makes sense that soaking in a bath of sea minerals will help to nourish, cleanse, and rejuvenate the cells in your skin.

Just as saltwater cleanses your skin, salt air opens, refreshes, and cleanses the breathing passages. This is why being at the seashore is so good for your lungs. Try practicing one of my deep–breathing techniques as you relax in your bath.

MORNING COLD SPLASH AND RUB

This Morning Cold Splash is an excellent way to wake yourself up before going for a brisk walk. It promotes the circulation and stimulates the systems of elimination. It is very beneficial if practiced regularly.

Be sure that your body temperature is warm before performing the Morning Cold Splash. Go directly from your warm bed, before early morning chill sets in.

Do the Cold Splash quickly, so that it doesn't take more than a few minutes. Sit in the empty tub with the stopper in place. Turn on the cold water and use your hands to splash it all over your body, washing first the arms and legs, then the abdomen, then the chest and back. Rub the skin with your hands as you splash water over your body. Us a brush to reach your back if you cannot reach it otherwise.

Leave the tub and dry yourself quickly with a coarse towel. Finish by rubbing with your hands until your skin is dry and smooth and you are glowing from the friction and the reaction to the cold water. At the end of this bath, you should feel warmth and comfort throughout your body.

EVENING "YOUTH BATH"

The cold sitz bath is often called a "youth bath" because of its rejuvenating effect. It stimulates the organs of elimination and reproduction. Taken just before bedtime, a cold sitz bath will produce a soothing and relaxing effect by drawing the blood away from the head and into the lower abdominal organs.

Be sure your body is warm before taking a cold sitz bath. Fill your bathtub shallowly with six to nine inches of cold water directly from the tap. Cover your shoulders and back with a towel, step into the tub, and, without hesitation, sit down. Keep your feet out of the water by resting them on the end of the tub or on an improvised footrest such as an inverted dishpan, so that only your "sitz" is covered by the water. Count slowly to sixty–the equivalent of one minute. You should notice a strong reaction, with the sensation of cold being followed by a feeling of warmth. Carefully rise from the tub, dry yourself with a coarse towel to warm the skin, then wrap yourself in a towel or robe for warmth, or get into bed and relax.

As you become accustomed to the cold water, you can gradually increase the sitting time, first to a count of 120, or two minutes, and then to 180.

SOOTHING "HOT SEAT" BATH

The hot sitz bath relaxes and warms the body, especially before bedtime. It relieves pain and inflammation in the pelvic organs, and is helpful for rectal problems. Later in the book on page 219 I will give a special recipe for a hot sitz bath to relieve menstrual discomfort.

Follow the directions for the cold sitz bath, except use water as hot as you can stand. Sit in the hot sitz bath for ten to fifteen minutes. Dry off with a coarse towel, then wrap yourself in a robe or get into bed to keep warm.

STRESS–REDUCTION BATH

Stress puts a tremendous strain on both the nervous system and the immune system, and can produce a state of mental and physical exhaustion. As the aromatic fumes of the essential oils in the Stress–Reduction Bath envelop you, they will help to strengthen and revive your nervous system. At the same time, they will relax your body and soothe away your anxieties.

>   6 drops basil essential oil
>   6 drops rosemary essential oil
>   6 drops chamomile essential oil

Add the essential oils to a hot bath. Lie back in the water and inhale the wonderful fragrance. Soak for twenty minutes, allowing the water to cool and bring your body back to normal temperature. Dry off vigorously with a coarse towel, wrap yourself in a warm robe, and prepare for a good night's sleep.

INSPIRATION BATH

The essential oils in the inspiration bath work together to create a euphoric, self–nurturing mood that will help you affirm your resolve to take better care of yourself. Eventually, you will come to associate these scents with feeling of self–love and well–being. Essence of rose is traditionally associated with love.

> Lavender essential oil
> Clary sage essential oil
> Rose essential oil (or blended rose oil)

To a hot bath, add six drops of each of the essential oils. Relax and inhale the fumes, allowing them to put you in a dreamy mood. Soak for twenty minutes as the water gradually cools. Dry yourself with a coarse towel and prepare for bed.

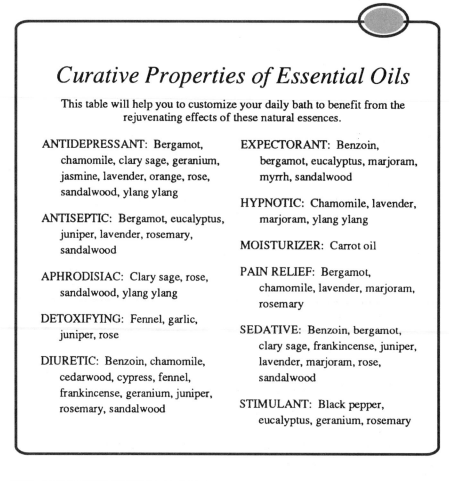

Curative Properties of Essential Oils

This table will help you to customize your daily bath to benefit from the rejuvenating effects of these natural essences.

ANTIDEPRESSANT: Bergamot, chamomile, clary sage, geranium, jasmine, lavender, orange, rose, sandalwood, ylang ylang

ANTISEPTIC: Bergamot, eucalyptus, juniper, lavender, rosemary, sandalwood

APHRODISIAC: Clary sage, rose, sandalwood, ylang ylang

DETOXIFYING: Fennel, garlic, juniper, rose

DIURETIC: Benzoin, chamomile, cedarwood, cypress, fennel, frankincense, geranium, juniper, rosemary, sandalwood

EXPECTORANT: Benzoin, bergamot, eucalyptus, marjoram, myrrh, sandalwood

HYPNOTIC: Chamomile, lavender, marjoram, ylang ylang

MOISTURIZER: Carrot oil

PAIN RELIEF: Bergamot, chamomile, lavender, marjoram, rosemary

SEDATIVE: Benzoin, bergamot, clary sage, frankincense, juniper, lavender, marjoram, rose, sandalwood

STIMULANT: Black pepper, eucalyptus, geranium, rosemary

TRANQUILITY BATH

Hot water is very enervating. Combined with the aromatic oils in this Tranquility Bath, it will help to calm and relax you after a busy day. Lavender and chamomile oils sooth away tension, lift the mood, and prepare you for sleep. Marjoram oil has an antispasmodic effect on tight, stressed–out muscles, and deepens the relaxation provided by the other oils.

Draw a hot bath and then add each of the following essential oils:

> 7 drops of lavender essential oil
> 10 drops chamomile essential oil
> 5 drops of marjoram essential oil

Lie back and feel the fumes penetrate your lungs and your skin. After your bath, douse yourself with a cool–to–cold sponge to close the pores and send the heat back to the center of your body. You will find this cool sponging very relaxing. Don't worry; it will not wake you up.

DEEP-HEAT BATH

Draw a very hot bath, then add each of the following essential oils:

> 10 drops eucalyptus essential oil
> 8 drops rosemary essential oil
> 5 drops sandalwood essential oil

The hot water helps to relax your muscles, and these essential oils are all beneficial for soothing your body after exercise. Eucalyptus oil is good for aching joints and muscles, and for skin problems and chapped skin. It is also used as an antiseptic inhalant, and the vapor helps clear the respiratory passages. Rosemary oil is a nervous–system stimulant. It is used as a tonic for the heart and to enhance liver functions. Hot compresses of rosemary oil are used for the aches and pains of rheumatism. Sandalwood oil cleanses and moisturizes the skin. Its lovely aroma is used in India to induce a meditative state.

Soak in this bath for twenty minutes, inhale the fumes, and feel them clearing your mind and your breathing passages, allowing the essential oils to work their magic.

CHAPARRAL DETOXIFYING BATH

A chaparral soak cleanses and detoxifies the blood, kidneys, liver, lymph, and thymus gland. Because chaparral is a powerful detoxifying agent, it helps to minimize cleansing reactions. Many people report that they feel "like new" after a chaparral bath, thanks to its restorative and deep–cleansing action.

Chaparral promotes immune–system functioning and fights bacteria and viruses. It contains a substance called NDGA, which prevents harmful oxidative processes that can lead to aging of the tissues.

Prepare a strong batch of chaparral bath tea at least one hour ahead of time, as follows:

> 4 tablespoons dried chaparral herb
> 1 quart purified water

Boil the water, remove from the heat, add the chaparral, and steep, covered, for one hour. Add the entire batch of chaparral tea (with the herb strained out) to a medium–to–hot bath. Soak in the tub for about twenty minutes, then dry quickly, wrap in a warm robe or towel, and lie down. Because chaparral flushes toxins out of the tissues so efficiently, it is a good idea to rest for ten to twenty minutes after your soak.

OPTIMISM BATH

Draw a warm bath and add five drops each of the essential oils of rose, rose geranium, lavender, and orange. Soak for at least twenty minutes to calm and heal troubled emotions or stress

I came across this bath one night when I was deeply dpressed over a broken romance, and could not get to sleep. It was too late to call a friend, get a massage, or go to the movies; so I consulted my reference books and came up with this combination of essential oils. I even dabbed a bit of the oil on my temples, and also made up the Easy Steam (described on page 152) and let the scented fumes fill the bathroom while I soaked in my bath. My mood improved dramatically.

Rose has an age–old reputation for healing the heart, and is traditionally associated with love. There are many varieties of rose essential oils, usually blended because pure rose oil is so expensive. Lavender is also soothing for the emotions, and orange oil has an antidepressant effect, helping to lift the mood.

CLEOPATRA'S MILK BATH

Milk has a well–deserved reputation for promoting a beautiful complexion, when used *externally*. It is excellent for general skin care, and smoothes dry, tired skin. This is the only use of milk that will be recommended during the 21–Day Program!

Simmer half a cup of barley in one quart of water, in a covered pot, for three hours. Prepare a larger quantity if you like, storing the extra barley water in your refrigerator. If you do not have time to simmer the barley, you can use half a cup of Rejuvelac instead.

Make one–fourth cup of almond meal by grinding whole raw almonds in a coffee grinder or blender. Combine the almond meal with one–fourth cup of oatmeal. Tie the mixture securely in a washcloth or cheesecloth. Fill your bathtub with warm water and add the bag of meal. Add three cups of milk along with half a cup of the cooked liquid from the barley; warm these liquids if necessary, so they will not cool the bathwater. Soak in this luxurious bath for twenty to thirty minutes, then finish off with a cold sponging or a cold shower. Wrap yourself in a towel and enjoy the feeling of cleanliness and youthfulness that this bath imparts to the skin.

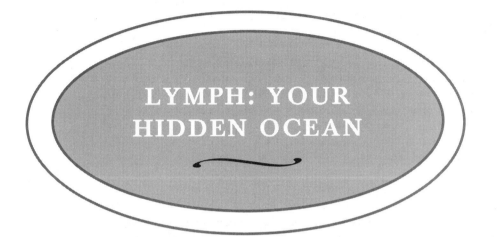

LYMPH: YOUR HIDDEN OCEAN

*A*s you relax in your cleansing and beautifying baths, remember that the interior of your body is also bathed in fluid. Much of this "inner ocean" is lymphatic fluid. Perhaps the only occasion you have had to be aware of your lymph system is when you had a sore throat or other infection, and felt enlarged lymph nodes in your neck or armpit or groin. These little pea–shaped organs are part of a network of delicate vessels throughout your body that transport the lymphatic fluid.

Lymph is a clear or milky fluid that originates in the blood capillaries, leaking out into the spaces between the cells. Inside the cells, fluids serve to transport nourishment and carry away wastes. Each cell is surrounded by a permeable membrane that allows materials to pass through to the outside. The fluid that bathes the outside of the cells is the lymph. Waste materials pass out of the cells, and out of the bloodstream through the capillary walls, and are eventually picked up by the lymph vessels. After traveling a short distance, these lymph vessels enter lymph nodes. The major lymph nodes are concentrated in the groin, armpits, neck, chest, and abdomen. Within specialized compartments in the lymph nodes are found different white cells, such as lymphocytes and macrophages, which have important functions in the immune system, protecting your body from infection and foreign materials. The lymphocytes circulate throughout the lymph system and attack invading organisms. When your body is fighting an infection, the lymph nodes become swollen near the site of the infection, as the bacteria are carried to the nodes, where they are engulfed and gobbled up by the macrophages. The lymph nodes also contain webbed areas that filter the lymph, removing foreign materials. After the lymph has been filtered, it leaves the lymph node, carrying the freshly cleaned lymph out the other side. The lymph vessels have valves, which allow the fluid to flow in only one direction, toward the heart. The lymph flow rejoins the bloodstream at the base of the neck, where the largest lymphatic collecting vessel, the thoracic duct, empties its lymph into the internal jugular vein to mix with the blood.

Normal lymph is a watery fluid, and it must remain at the proper consistency in order to move readily through its vessels. Certain kinds of debris and toxic materials cause the lymph to become thick or mucoidlike in consistency.

As you might expect, the lymph system has a direct impact on the appearance and condition of your skin. When the lymph system becomes clogged, it is not able to carry the impurities away as readily for excretion, placing a burden on the other organs of elimination; and so, many of the waste products end up being trapped or excreted by the skin. Similarly, cellulite deposits tend to form when toxins carried by stagnant lymph get lodged in fatty accumulations just beneath the skin.

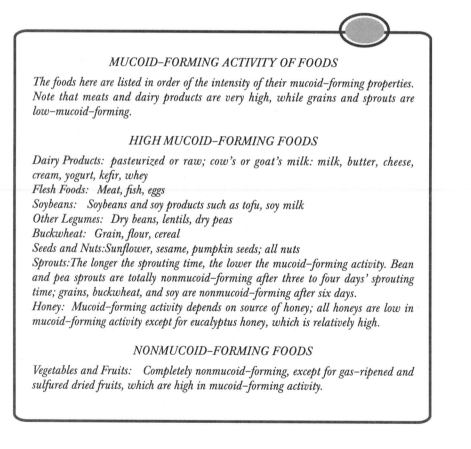

MUCOID-FORMING ACTIVITY OF FOODS

The foods here are listed in order of the intensity of their mucoid-forming properties. Note that meats and dairy products are very high, while grains and sprouts are low-mucoid-forming.

HIGH MUCOID-FORMING FOODS

Dairy Products: pasteurized or raw; cow's or goat's milk: milk, butter, cheese, cream, yogurt, kefir, whey
Flesh Foods: Meat, fish, eggs
Soybeans: Soybeans and soy products such as tofu, soy milk
Other Legumes: Dry beans, lentils, dry peas
Buckwheat: Grain, flour, cereal
Seeds and Nuts:Sunflower, sesame, pumpkin seeds; all nuts
Sprouts:The longer the sprouting time, the lower the mucoid-forming activity. Bean and pea sprouts are totally nonmucoid-forming after three to four days' sprouting time; grains, buckwheat, and soy are nonmucoid-forming after six days.
Honey: Mucoid-forming activity depends on source of honey; all honeys are low in mucoid-forming activity except for eucalyptus honey, which is relatively high.

NONMUCOID-FORMING FOODS

Vegetables and Fruits: Completely nonmucoid-forming, except for gas-ripened and sulfured dried fruits, which are high in mucoid-forming activity.

KEEPING YOUR LYMPH CLEAN AND CLEAR

Every aspect of my Cleansing and Rejuvenation Program is designed to promote the proper functioning of your lymphatic system. Let's begin by looking again at the food you eat.

You may have heard some discussion of so-called "mucus–forming" foods. This term is something of a misnomer. Clear, slippery mucus is a normal secretion of the mucous membranes. The sticky mucoid material that can clog up the lymph system is not produced by the mucous membranes; rather, it is an accumulation of incompletely broken–down nutrients and waste products that tend to thicken the lymph and make it harder for it to move through the body and cleanse the tissues. Foods vary greatly in their tendency to form mucoid material, with foods high in protein and fat having the greatest mucoid–forming power. The diet in your Cleansing and Rejuvenation Program emphasizes non–mucoid–forming foods, such as vegetables and fruits.

Another factor that influences lymph function is the condition of your colon. When the colon is clear and its walls unlined with waste deposits, the colon wall is able to absorb mucoid material from the lymph for excretion. When you are constipated or the walls of your colon are caked with toxic wastes, mucoid material begins to back up into the lymphatic system. In the second week of this program, you will begin a gentle process of colon cleansing that will help to drain mucoid material out of your lymph system and keep it clear and clean.

Exercise is another very important factor in keeping your lymph clear. Whereas your blood is moved through the body by the pumping action of your heart, the lymph system depends on the contraction of the muscles surrounding the vessels to keep it moving along. Muscular contractions increase pressure within the system, causing the valves to close; when pressure decreases, the valves open and the lymph flows. When the body is not moving, the lymph in the arms, legs, and head does not move measurably. With activity, drainage of the lymph system increases tenfold. Some kinds of exercise are better than others for moving the lymph through the system. All vigorous exercise, such as brisk walking with strongly swinging arms, is beneficial in moving the lymph. Be sure to regularly practice the Lymph Cleansing Warm–up Exercises on page 118.

FOOT SOAKS

Foot soaks are an excellent way to stimulate lymphatic function, especially in the lower lymphatic vessels which tend to get sluggish and clogged because of the effects of gravity. Soaking your feet helps to open the pores and draw the toxins out of the lymph system through the skin. The Romans knew the value of bathing the feet in the waters of their healing springs, and at the great French spas, footbaths were the prescribed treatment for arthritis. The effects of footbaths are aided by specific minerals or herbs added to the water, and by the temperature of the water itself.

"Hot Foot" Soak

Mustard has been valued for centuries in both Eastern and Western medicine for its ability to stimulate blood and body–fluid circulation and break up stagnation. Its effects are powerful, so be careful not to use more than the recommended amount of mustard powder.

This foot soak will cause you to sweat profusely as the effects of the mustard promote the expulsion of wastes from your entire system.

In a gallon bucket or small tub, dissolve three tablespoons of mustard powder in very hot water, as hot as you can stand. Soak your feet for twenty minutes. Mustard powder is a powerful rubefacient, causing the skin to redden as it dilates the blood vessels near the surface of the skin, bringing more blood to the area. It also draws lymph to the surface, helping to flush it of toxins and waste materials. Miraculously, mustard foot soaks have been used successfully to relieve the pain of earache, tooth abscess, and sinusitis by drawing the body fluids to the surface of the feet.

Father Kneipp's Foot Bath

Father Kneipp was one of the modern pioneers in the therapeutic uses of water. This hot–and–cold contrast foot bath is considered an excellent treatment for colds, sinusitis, headaches, poor circulation, neuritis, and congested abdominal organs. Try it the next time you are feeling congestion or sluggishness anywhere in your body.

Fill one small tub or gallon bucket with hot water, and a second tub with cold water. The water in each tub should be eight to twelve inches deep. Place your feet in the hot tub for three to five minutes, then switch to the cold tub for thirty seconds. Repeat this procedure twice.

As with any alternating hot–and–cold bath or shower, this footbath is very invigorating. You will find it wakes up your whole body and leaves you feeling energized.

LYMPHATIC MASSAGE

After your foot soak, an excellent way to continue lymphatic stimulation is through massage. You have already learned how to do dry brush massaging on page 144. Skin brushing is one of the best ways known to stimulate the expulsion of mucoid material and other obstructions from the lymphatic system, and for correcting inflammations of the lymph nodes. Skin brushing works hand in hand with colon cleansing to keep the lymphatic system clear. Now, I am going to show you how to do a lymphatic self–massage in order to stimulate lymph flow in your lower body. Remember that the lymph flows toward the heart–up from the feet and down from the head.

Lower–Body Lymphatic Massage

Massage one leg at a time. Using one or two hands, begin by massaging at the base of each toe and between the toes. Massage gently in a circular motion; imagine yourself loosening the toxins and debris from all the tiny lymph vessels between your toes.

After you have gently massaged the base of each toe, stroke upward with both hands, drawing the lymph up and toward the ankles with a gentle, feathery, upward stroking motion. Move up to the ankle; gently massage in a circular motion all around the ankle, and then lightly stoke upward, drawing the lymph up the calf until you get to the knee.

Massage with both hands all around the knee, over the lymph nodes behind the knee, and around the kneecap, in circular motions. Use light pressure; this is the best way to stimulate the lymph. Remember that the lymph vessels are close to the surface of the skin.

Draw the lymph up along the thighs, using the fingertips or the palms of the hands. At the back of the thigh, massage gently at the base of the buttock, in a gentle circular motion; this is one of the areas where the toxic waste of cellulite tends to accumulate.

Stroke upward, along the thigh, and bring it all around and back into the groin. After you have completed one leg, work on the other leg.

In the groin area, work on both sides at once. Stroke upward and diagonally across the groin area with the flat of the hand on each side, moving the hands toward each other so they come together over the abdomen. Repeat this upward stroking all along the groin area; there are many lymph nodes in this area.

As you stroke gently upward and into the abdominal area, picture all the debris and waste being moved along, to be absorbed and eliminated through your colon.

When you do a lymphatic massage, you may notice that some areas react painfully to pressure. Most people, for example, if they press hard between their breasts, will feel a very sensitive spot. This is one of the areas where lymph congestion can produce tenderness. If you find such a sensitive spot, do not be afraid to touch it; continue to gently massage it with a light, circular motion, and then, with a feathery touch, move it onward–up from the legs, down from the head. As you progress in your Cleansing and Rejuvenation Program, you will notice that there is less and less lymphatic congestion and that you have fewer sensitive spots.

Spend about ten minutes on the lymphatic massage. Proper lymphatic functioning produces clear, glowing skin; and, because it is a vital part of your immune system, it helps to promote your resistance to disease.

Upper–Body Lymph Massage

This gentle upper–body self–massage, which you will perform on the evening of Day 10, helps to flush congested lymph out of the extremities and toward the heart, where it joins the main lymph drainage of the body. Combined with skin brushing and detoxifying baths, lymph massage also assists in rejuvenating the complexion.

Begin your massage at the neck, under the chin, in the areas where you may have sometimes noticed swollen lymph glands. Massage with the fingertips from ear to ear in a gentle circular motion, then gently stroke from the ears under the chin toward the center. Now, with your fingertips, gently

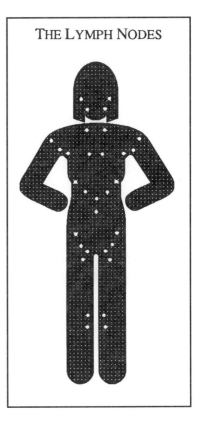

THE LYMPH NODES

stroke downward, from under the chin down the neck. Use these gentle downward stroking movements all around the neck, moving the lymph from beneath the chin and the base of the skull down into the top of your chest.

Next, using your left hand, work on the right arm, beginning at the wrist. Use your fingers to repeatedly smooth and stroke the inside of the arm, from the wrist up to the inner elbow. When you reach the inside of the elbow, gently massage with a circular motion, then continue with a light, feathery, stroking movement up the inside of the arm to the underarm. In the armpit area, gently squeeze with thumb and fingers, releasing the lymph and moving it up and out of the arm. This is another area where many lymph nodes are located, and where you may have noticed swelling when you have been sick. Stroke from the armpit up over the top of the right breast, using light, feathery strokes to bring the lymph out of the armpit and around toward the center of the chest. Guide the lymph from the right shoulder, the right arm area, and the neck, all down toward the middle of the chest.

Now, use the right hand and repeat this process, bringing the lymph up the left arm and into the armpit. Concentrate a little longer on the left side, to work the lymph out of the armpit and along the extensive lymph drainage around the heart. Draw it all in toward the center of the chest, into the area between the breasts. Now, rub in a gentle circular motion between the breasts. It is quite possible that you will feel some tenderness in this area; this simply means that there is some lymph congestion here. Do not be alarmed; just continue to gently massage, and over time the congestion will begin to be relieved. Now, massage beneath the breasts, about an inch or so below each breast, stroking gently around the bottom of the breasts toward the middle, bringing it all down into the abdomen. Stroke gently downward all the way across your chest beneath your breasts, moving the lymph into the abdomen, where the waste will be eliminated by the colon.

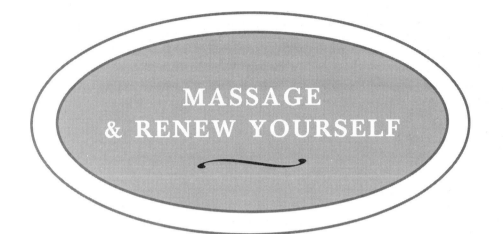

MASSAGE & RENEW YOURSELF

Massage is a remarkably effective and deeply pleasurable method for moving fresh, rejuvenating fluids into the cells and pushing the stale, toxin–laden fluids out. At the same time, massage is also a powerful tool for managing stress, which can age even the best–nourished complexion and mar the look of vitality in even the best–exercised body.

As we saw in the last chapter, it is also a powerful tool for keeping the lymphatic system clean and clear.

For many people, the idea of massage summons up images of sleazy "massage parlors" or self–indulgent pampering exclusively for the idle rich. Our society still retains many of its puritanical attitudes about the human body, clinging to the belief that anything that feels good cannot really be good for the health or the character.

I would like to dispel such negative, fearful ideas about massage once and for all. For me, massage is an essential part of my health–maintenance program. It is an effective way of releasing the stress that builds up in my daily life, and it is a very important way for me to take care of myself. If I cannot express love for myself and take care of my own body, then how can I love and take care of other people, both professionally and in my personal life?

I am not unique in this attitude. Many successful sports figures, entertainers, business people, and politicians depend on massage to improve their performance, keep them youthful and attractive, and relieve their stress. Lee Iacocca, after his retirement from the Ford Motor Company, continued to receive massages from the company masseur. Members of the U.S. Olympic

Team were given massages after competing in their events in Calgary, Canada, and Seoul, Korea. Celebrities like Bette Midler, Tina Turner, Madonna, Bob Hope, Bruce Springsteen, and Luciano Pavarotti all rely on regular massage to keep them fit, youthful, and able to manage the stress of their hectic public lives.

The use of touch to soothe physical and emotional pain is a built–in response in the human organism. Even animals lick their wounds and groom one another. Massage has a long history in the healing arts. A Chinese medical treatise recorded the use of massage as early as 3000 B.C. and the ancient Hindu literature described its therapeutic value around 1800 B.C. In ancient Greece, Hippocrates, the father of Western medicine, taught that physicians must be experienced in the healing art of rubbing. In Rome, Julius Caesar received daily massages for his neuralgia. During the Middle Ages, massage (and bathing) fell out of favor as the church encouraged a general disdain for "fleshly indulgences." With the rebirth of interest in bodily health during the Renaissance, massage again grew in popularity and began to develop as a science. Many prominent physicians subsequently included massage as part of their repertoire of healing techniques.

In this century, massage has repeatedly come in and out of fashion. During World War I, it was used to treat wounded soldiers. The human potential movement in the 1970's brought new attention to the healing power of touch. Today, massage is becoming very respectable once again, and competent professional massage therapists are available in ever-increasing numbers.

HOW MASSAGE HELPS TO KEEP YOU YOUNG

My Inner Beauty Program would not be as effective without the catalytic effects of total body massage. Many people think that I look much younger than my years. I attribute much of my youthful appearance and clear complexion to massage. For me, massage has pulled all the other aspects of my self–care program together into a unique, rejuvenating combination. I first started receiving massage when I was doing competitive swimming in grammar school. I noticed that the older, more advanced swimmers were having regular massage, and so I tried it, too. I discovered that if I had a massage after a strenuous workout, I would recover faster, my pre–competition tension would be relieved, and I would be able to swim farther and faster. Later, when I became involved in dance, I used massage to help stretch my muscles and prevent injuries. I then began to study yoga, and noticed that yoga postures served as a sort of self–massage. Like massage, yoga also helped to promote my own body awareness.

Massage is a vital part of staying young. It supports the cleansing and nourishing of the cells by stimulating circulation—of lymph, of blood, and of energy. Massage causes the blood vessels to dilate, so that circulation is improved and congestion is relieved. It temporarily raises the red blood–cell count, by moving sedentary cells into circulation, thereby increasing the oxygen–carrying capacity of the blood. With increased oxygenation of the cells, the metabolic rate is increased, wastes are broken down more completely, and the calories in your food are burned more efficiently. Massage also helps to push the lymph along in its channels, delivering nutrients, hastening the elimination of waste, and keeping the immune system health.

Oriental healing systems teach that massage affects the energy system in the body that flows through channels known as meridians. This meridian energy is the basis of the Chinese science of acupuncture, which holds that illness is a result of blockage or stagnation of this energy flow. In acupuncture, sterile needles are inserted into specific points along the meridians to stimulate energy flow. Oriental systems of massage, such as acupressure or shiatsu, rather than using needles, simply apply pressure to these very same points to unblock the flow of energy.

Massage helps you to get the greatest possible benefit from your exercise program. By stimulating the circulation of blood and lymph, massage helps to bring fuel—oxygen and nutrients—to the muscles. At the same time, it carries away metabolic waste. Lactic acid, which is produced as a metabolic by–product of exercise, causes muscle soreness and a feeling of fatigue. Massage helps to move this lactic acid out of the muscles, speeding recovery time after strenuous exercise.

Massage also preserves muscle tone. If injury, illness, or an overly demanding schedule force you to be physically inactive for some time, massage can help to compensate for the lack of exercise. I became aware of the toning and conditioning benefits of massage during the years when an increasingly busy professional life caused me to drop exercise from my daily activities. If it weren't for the regular massages I had during this period, I probably would not have maintained the muscle tone that I still enjoy today.

Because it promotes body awareness, massage can also help to prevent injuries. So often we tend to disregard the messages from our bodies. We may push ourselves beyond the limit of some part of our body that is tense or sore or weak. Having a regular massage helps you tune in to these problem areas so that you can work with them before they break down or become injured.

If you should happen to be injured, massage also helps to promote rapid healing. It reduces swelling by carrying fluid away from the injured area. It keeps muscle fibers from developing adhesions or fibrosis. Massage has even been shown to speed the healing of fractures by influencing metabolism and encouraging the retention of minerals needed for the bone repair.

For me, the psychological benefits are probably the most important aspect of massage. We live in a society that is starved for touch. It is a perfectly natural thing to touch a child, a friend, or even a stranger to comfort or soothe them. Sometimes a wordless hand on the shoulder, a hug or a stroke on the back can be the most healing thing we can do for another person. Research at the University of Miami Medical School showed that premature infants who were massaged for fifteen minutes three times a day gained weight 47 percent faster than babies who were left alone in their incubators, as was the usual practice. The massaged infants showed more rapid development of their nervous systems, and were able to leave the hospital six days earlier than other premature infants who were not massaged. Skin–to–skin touch is essential for all babies, premature or not. Infants receiving more touch have been shown to have a six–month advantage in their mental development. As a result of such findings, American parents are now learning techniques for massaging their infants–an activity that is a natural part of child care in many other parts of the world.

Adults as well as infants require physical touch. I find that getting a massage is one of the most effective ways to nurture and take care of myself. Many people seek out sexual contacts simply because they need to be touched, and do not realize that they can get touch in other ways as well.

Anita, one of my clients, was typical of such people. A successful artist, she worked alone in her studio, and she lived alone as well. During the time I worked with Anita on a cleansing program, she confided to me that she was having a lot of trouble with her relationships. She would get sexually involved with one man after another, and never seemed to find the love or satisfaction she was looking for. As we talked, it became clear that she was really hungry for touch. I suggested that she try massage, and she discovered that receiving a massage once a week helped her to place sex in the proper perspective and enabled her to be more discriminating in her relationships.

For me, massage is essential for stress management. Stress can have a very aging effect on the appearance, causing furrowing of the brow and worry lines around the mouth and between the eyebrows. I remember one massage therapist who would always point out when I was frowning. I had never realized until then how much tension I was holding in my face. A very important part of stress management is being aware of your stress–warning signals. Being touched by another person helps you to tune into every part of your body and to see where you are holding stress and tension. Over time, such stress held in the body can lead to real physical symptoms. Massage helps call attention to these warning signs before they reach the danger point.

Massage is becoming so widely accepted as a stress reliever today that many major corporations, such as Apple Computer and AT&T, now sponsor regular in–office massages for their employees. In cities across the United States, therapists are providing "on–site" massages that generally take about fifteen minutes.

Relieving stress through massage will help to keep you on track as you follow the 21–Day Cleansing and Rejuvenation Program. Sometimes it is just what is needed to break through old stress patterns and allow your body and mind to experience the dramatic benefits of the sweeping lifestyle changes you are undertaking. A client of mine, a busy executive named Alan, is a perfect example of the hard–driving, Type–A personality. He was having trouble with his digestion, and he was constipated most of the time. Although he denied it initially, it was obvious to me that a great deal of his problem was due to stress. He worked hard at changing his diet, took all the recommended supplements, adhered faithfully to his exercise, and cooperated in the cleansing program, but he was still holding a lot of stress in his body, particularly in his abdominal organs. Finally, I persuaded Alan to set up a series of appointments for massage. For the first time, Alan allowed someone to do something for him, rather than insisting on controlling what was happening to him. With regular weekly massage sessions, Alan finally learned how to let go and relax. He began to respond better to the cleansing program, and he also began to understand what I meant when I suggested he use his exercise period as a time to relax and breathe and open himself up to the beauty of the outdoors, rather than feeling compelled to push himself through a strenuous daily regimen. All the components of his cleansing program began to fall into place once he learned to relax and tune in to the stress signals his body was sending him.

I often find that tension held in the abdomen can be the principal cause of problems with digestion and elimination. Stress can cause clenching of the muscles along the intestinal tract, inhibiting peristalsis and preventing proper digestion and bowel movement. Massage is a great tool for helping people to recognize these muscular holding patterns and learn to release them.

WHICH MASSAGE IS RIGHT FOR YOU?

Essentially, massage can be divided into four main categories: Swedish, Oriental or shiatsu, reflexology, and sports massage. Each type of massage is used for different purposes, and has a different "feel." It is very common for massage therapists to combine elements of different techniques into a more eclectic approach.

My own personal health–maintenance program includes at least one professional massage per week. Every other week, I receive an eclectic bodywork type of massage that works at a very deep tissue level, not only moving the blood and lymph but also producing intense emotional release. On the alternating weeks, I have a Swedish type of massage that helps to keep my lymph moving, relaxes me and relieves my stress, and is wonderfully nurturing. Whenever I am out of balance or feeling emotionally vulnerable, I may have an additional Swedish massage during the week.

Swedish massage, introduced by Peter Ling of Sweden in the nineteenth century, combines traditional techniques brought back from China with a Western understanding of anatomy and physiology. Swedish massage works with the body's muscular and skeletal structure to promote circulation, soothe the nervous system, and promote a feeling of well–being. It consists of long, gliding strokes, and a variety of kneading, friction, squeezing, tapping, and shaking movements. Swedish massage is given on a table, with the client partially or completely undressed, since the massage therapist works directly on the bare skin, using oil for lubrication. Because Swedish massage concentrates on promoting circulation of blood and lymph, it is ideally suited to the whole–body cleansing of the 21–Day Program. You will also find it wonderfully relaxing. A less vigorous variant of Swedish massage, known as Esalen massage, uses gentle, rhythmic movements that many people find to be a good introduction to the nurturing, relaxing benefits of massage.

Shiatsu massage, also known as acupressure, is an Oriental technique based on the acupuncture theory of meridian energy. By applying pressure rather than needles to specific points along the meridians, this form of massage is believed to unblock the circulation of the life energy, helping to promote self–healing and prevent illness. Therapists who use these Oriental techniques work with their fingers, hands, elbows, and knees on points along the energy pathways. The deep pressure of shiatsu massage may feel painful when applied to sore, tense muscles; while some people enjoy this intense stimulation, others may find it too much for them. Oriental massage tends to produce an energized feeling rather than relaxation, and is helpful for relieving tension in specific areas of the body. It is usually performed on a mat on the floor, with the client wearing loose, comfortable clothing.

Reflexology is a form of acupressure that concentrates on the feet, and sometimes the hands. It is based on the theory that every organ, muscle, and gland in the body corresponds to a specific area on the feet. By manipulating the appropriate part of the feet, the masseur can relieve tension in the corresponding distant part. I have found, for example, that clients with elimination or digestion problems are able to relax in their abdominal organs when I massage the colon point in the middle of the sole of the foot. Introduced relatively recently in the early 1900's, reflexology is based on ancient Chinese, Japanese, and Egyptian techniques. You can do this particular kind of massage for yourself, or a massage therapist can give you a reflexology foot or hand massage while you are lying on a table or sitting in a reclining chair. Try massaging your feet as a pleasant, effective way to induce relaxation.

Sports massage is a rapidly growing sub–specialty in the Untied States today. It caters specifically to serious athletes, but is becoming increasingly popular among amateurs as well. Sports massage consists of a combination of Swedish–massage strokes and pressure–point techniques derived from shiatsu, as well as specific manipulations to prevent injury, improve performance, and aid recovery. If you are actively engaged in a sport that places stress on certain joints or muscles, you may find that sports massage, focused on those parts of your body, can be a valuable part of your training program. Sports massage tends to be brisk, vigorous, and more energizing than a relaxing full–body Swedish massage.

Other forms of massage include Rolfing, which works on deep tissues to release tension patterns stored in the muscles and joints, and provides a release of emotions held in the body. Bodywork techniques such as the Trager and Feldenkreis methods and Polarity therapy use movement and manipulation to balance the body energies and release physical and emotional patterns. These emotional–release forms of massage are really in the realm of psychotherapy. While they can be enormously effective, they are actually beyond the scope of the 21–Day Cleansing and Rejuvenation Program, which emphasizes the circulation–enhancing and stress-relieving benefits of massage. If you are accustomed to one of these body techniques, please feel free to continue with it as your massage therapy of choice.

WATER MASSAGE

At physical therapy centers and European health spas, massage and treatments with water are an inseparable part of the natural healing programs. While massage was largely ignored in American health spas until recently, the healing effects of hydrotherapy, or water treatment, have always been recognized. The external application of water affects many of the same systems as massage. Like massage, hydrotherapy influences the circulation of the blood, soothes the nervous system, and helps the eliminative function of the skin.

You may be surprised at the powerful effect cold water has as a hydrotherapy treatment. Cold water applied to the skin actually stimulates circulation throughout the system. As with massage, cold water applications mobilize sluggish blood cells throughout the body, moving them into circulation and temporarily increasing both the red and white blood cell counts. The initial effect of cold water applications is to chill the skin and drive the blood toward the center of the body, where the body's heat–regulating mechanism then produces a reaction, causing the blood to rush back to the surface, open the pores and capillaries, and release impurities through the skin in the form of perspiration. The Morning Cold Splash and Rub on page 154 is an excellent illustration of how this process works, as is the cold sitz bath, or "Youth Bath" on page 154. While the initial effect of these procedures is to produce chilling, a healthy body will rapidly react by producing the opposite effect, and a warm flushing suffuses the parts that have been exposed to the cold water.

A great way to warm up cold feet is to stimulate circulation in them through a reflex reaction to cold. Try walking barefoot in cold dewy grass or on wet stones, or even in the snow. Once you feel the flushing reaction, get into a warm place, cover up, and enjoy the tingling heat in your feet and toes.

EXPERIENCING MASSAGE

On Day 16, at the end of the cleansing phase of this program, you are scheduled to receive a professional massage that helps to promote the cleansing process and give you an added psychological boost. If possible, arrange for the massage therapist to come to your home, so that you can enjoy a relaxing day in your private spa environment.

I recommend a Swedish–type massage because of its great benefits for the circulation of blood and lymph, as well as the wonderful relaxation it induces. If you are very active athletically and tend to have problems in any particular part of your body, you may want to look for a massage therapist who is also familiar with sports massage.

Feel free to schedule additional massages if you wish. The more regularly you receive a massage, the greater are the benefits. Even after one session, however, you should notice a positive difference. You will probably feel marvelously relaxed immediately after your massage, although you may feel a little sluggish the day afterward, as toxins are being mobilized out of your system. To minimize such effects, be sure to drink several glasses of the Hydrating Drink or purified water right after your massage to stimulate lymph flow and carry away the freshly released toxins. Continue to drink water throughout the day, perhaps several glasses more than usual. If you do not feel an immediate improvement after one massage session, you many want to try a different therapist or a different kind of massage the next time.

If you are suffering from any medical problem, check with your physician

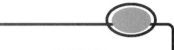

MASSAGE SELF–INSTRUCTION AIDS

Learn massage techniques by yourself or with a friend. I highly recommend these books:

The Magic of Massage *by Ouida West (Hastings)*

The Book of Massage *by Lucinda Lidell, et al. (Fireside)*

My favorite videotape, covering both Swedish and acupressure techniques, is Massage Your Mate, *available from Ozman Inc., 496 Hudson Street, Suite K-17, New York 10014.*

Another excellent videotape is Massage for Health *by Shari Belafonte (Healing Arts), widely available in video stores.*

before you receive a massage. Massage is not advised if you have a fever, an ulcer, cancer, high blood pressure, or a recent fracture or dislocation. If you have varicose veins, an infection, or recently torn tendons, ligaments, or muscles, do not have these sensitive areas massaged, and be sure to call them to the attention of the therapist. Pregnant women and people with heart disease or bone disease should check with their physician before getting a massage.

How to Choose A Massage Therapist

Your massage therapist will be providing a very personal service for you, and you want to be sure you will feel comfortable with the person you select. Begin by asking your friends if they have a favorite massage therapist. A personal referral helps to ensure that the therapist is ethical and experienced. Sometimes it can be difficult to differentiate the legitimate massage therapist among the listings in the telephone yellow pages or the classified ads in a newspaper. If there is an alternative publication in your area such as Common Ground, you will find qualified massage therapists listed there. You can also call the Chicago offices of the American Massage Therapy Association at (312) 761-AMTA for referrals to massage therapists in your area.

Some states require a license to practice massage therapy. If your state requires a license, make sure that your therapist has one. Ask what kind of training the therapist has had; ideally, select someone who has gone through an extensive formal training program, including the study of anatomy and physiology. Experience is just as important as training. I recommend that you look for a therapist who has been in practice for at least one year.

It is not unusual to feel self–conscious about your body, or anxious about what will happen, at your first session with a massage therapist. You may feel apprehensive about being naked, or about having a stranger touch you. A good massage therapist is sensitive to your feelings and will not push you to do anything that you don't want to. If you are not comfortable removing all your clothes, leave on your underwear. Once you are on the massage table, the therapist will drape you with sheets and towels, both to respect your modesty and to keep your body warm.

At your first meeting, the massage therapist should ask you about your physical condition and your personal needs. You will be asked whether you have any medical problems, are pregnant, on medication, or menstruating, and whether you have had any recent surgery. The answers to these questions will determine what kind of massage you will receive.

Do not hesitate to discuss the cost of the massage when you first call the therapist on the phone. In most parts of the country, rates generally average in the thirty–dollar to fifty–dollar range for a one–hour massage. If there is a massage school in you area, and you are willing to allow a beginner to work on you, call and inquire whether the school offers sessions with apprentices. The rates will be considerably lower.

While I recommend a professional massage on a regular, once a week basis, this is more than some people can afford. An alternative is to pay for a professional massage as often as you can, and on other weeks call on a friend. You may both need instruction to make the exchange of massage as beneficial as possible. See if massage classes are offered in your area. If you don't have time for a class, some excellent self–teaching materials are available. Exchanging massage with a mate or a friend can be a pleasant and meaningful way to share healing, loving energy. Not only is it wonderful to receive a massage, but it is a very satisfying experience to know how to give one to someone close to you.

MAKE YOUR OWN AROMATHERAPY MASSAGE OIL

Massaging the skin with essential oils is an ideal way to get the healing properties of aromatic plant essences into the body. The herbal essences are absorbed even more readily through the skin than through inhalation. Try rubbing some essential oil on the palm of your hand; you should be able to taste it in your mouth in a couple of minutes. The nurturing touch of massage enhances the relaxing, soothing, and stimulating properties of the oils themselves.

You can prepare your own massage oil to use regularly for all the massage activities in this program.

In an eight–ounce container, place the following vegetable oils, which will serve as the base for the essential oils:

> 3 ounces of olive oil
> 3 ounces of almond oil
> 2 ounces of peanut oil

Olive oil moisturizes and softens the skin, soothes irritation, and alleviates dryness of cuticles and nails. Almond oil is an excellent moisturizer that imparts its fragrance to many fine cosmetics. Peanut oil is believed to be very beneficial for the joints, and is used frequently in natural remedies applied externally for arthritis.

To the base mixture, add essential oils to make your own personalized massage oil formula. A good general–purpose combination is:

> 12 drops of eucalyptus oil
> 15 drops of lavender oil
> 15 drops of chamomile oil
> 12 drops of rosemary oil

These essential oils have a pleasant sedative effect, promote circulation, and relax the muscles. To make a mixture more personalized to your taste and needs, consult the chart Curative Properties of Essential Oils on page 156.

Varicose Veins. Prepare a small batch of the following special massage oil to help increase circulation and improve the tone of the veins.

> 1 ounce of olive oil
> 8 drops of cypress essential oil

Massage with this oil only above the area affected with varicose veins, never below—that is, massage between the varicosities and the heart. Use this oil only for those parts of your body, such as your legs, that have the varicose veins, and use your regular massage oil for the other body areas.

SELF-MASSAGE

While nothing can equal the relaxation and sense of being cared for that you derive from receiving a professional massage, you can experience many of the benefits of massage by doing it for yourself. Through self-massage, you can develop a better understanding of your own body. Because you are getting your own feedback, you will know exactly how much pressure to apply without causing pain, and you will discover what feels best to you. Self-massage allows you to tune in to areas where you are holding tension in your body, to relieve aching muscles and release energy blockages. Whenever you feel tense and under pressure, use these massage techniques, drawn from Swedish and Oriental massage, to relax and nurture yourself.

Anti-Gravity Facial Massage

Massaging your face on a slant board is particularly beneficial because the antigravity position brings the blood supply to the face, so this massage is beautifying as well as relaxing. You can use the same facial-massage techniques whenever you are under stress. In the privacy of your office, in the bathroom at work, or while commuting by bus, train, or car, you can do a one-minute version of this facial massage for a quick relaxer and youth restorer.

Set up the slant board as described on page 122. Relax for a few minutes in the antigravity position, with your feet above your head. Breathe in through your nostrils and out through pursed lips to calm and center yourself. Before you begin, dab a little massage oil or cream of your choice on your fingertips. If you have never been introduced to castor oil, this is a good time to try it; an occasional facial massage with castor oil is very rejuvenating to the skin. Castor oil is a popular folk remedy for all sorts of skin problems, and is an ingredient in many cosmetics because of its hydrating and soothing properties. You may also use your own massage oil or plain vegetable oil; see page 173 for some recommended oils for different skin types.

Now, with your fingertips, gently massage your temples in a circular motion. Move all around the temple area. If you find a sensitive spot, do not avoid it, but bring your attention to that spot and gently massage the tenderness away. Continue your conscious breathing as you feel the relaxation spread through the muscles of your face.

Next, use your fingertips to gently massage between your eyebrows in a circular motion. Then stroke your fingertips across your forehead, moving out from the center toward the temples. Use gentle but firm pressure, as much pressure as feels comfortable to you. Work your way up and down the forehead, stroking across in this manner, so that you cover the entire forehead. Then place the fingertips of each hand along the corresponding eyebrow and with firm but gentle pressure slide the fingertips from the eyebrows into the hairline. Cover the entire forehead with this sliding motion, to relax the forehead and smooth out the wrinkles in your brow.

Massage your cheeks by sliding the fingers upward on each side, from the chin up over the cheeks, out to the temples and into the hairline. Repeat this movement several times, covering the sides of the face completely. Then massage in a circular motion over the cheekbones, beginning below the outer corners of the eyes, moving across the cheek and down to the base of your nose. Massage in a circular motion back out and down to the hinge of the jaw. Spend some time massaging here, noticing any tender spots. Many people hold a lot of tension in the jaw.

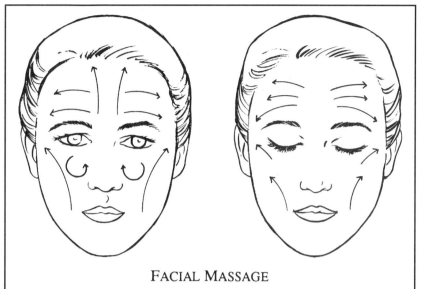

FACIAL MASSAGE

As you massage your face, feel the muscles relax and the blood flow into all the tissues, nourishing them and bringing a glow to your complexion. This facial massage is also helpful for freeing the sinuses of congestion.

Finish your facial massage by placing your thumbs under your chin and pulling them up, first on one side and then the other, along the jawline toward the ears. The longer you continue this alternate chin stroking, the greater will be the toning effect if you have a tendency to a sagging chin line.

Continue your facial massage for a full five minutes. Then, still lying on the slant board, use your fingertips to massage your scalp. Use the pads of the fingers, being careful not to damage the scalp with your nails. If you find tender spots, concentrate on those. Massage in a circular motion over the entire scalp, being sure to go all the way down to the neck and behind the ears. This scalp massage encourages hair growth and improves scalp problems. Keep up the scalp massage for two to three minutes. It is a very relaxing and pleasant way to enhance your natural beauty.

Quick Oriental Massage Remedies

Pressure–point massage techniques are derived from shiatsu and acupressure. During the 21–Day Program, you may experience some minor discomforts as your body is ridding itself of toxins. Try these massage remedies for drugless first–aid the next time you have the indicated problem.

HEADACHE Press your left thumb onto the back of your right hand, in the web of flesh between the base of the thumb and the bone that connects to the forefinger. Hold firmly for five seconds to two minutes, and you should feel your headache pain subside. This acupressure point was known in ancient times as the "Great Eliminator."

CONSTIPATION Move your left thumb just up from the Great Eliminator point, so that you are pressing with the thumb into the inside edge of metacarpal bone of the right index finger, just beyond the V where this bone meets the bone from the thumb. Hold this point firmly while attempting to move the bowels, to ease tension in the large intestine.

LOW ENERGY Massaging specific points in the abdomen and the chest is a great substitute for coffee, whenever you are groggy and want to stay awake–while driving, working, or dozing off at a

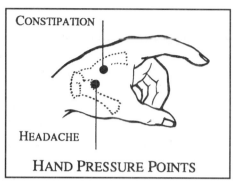

CONSTIPATION

HEADACHE

HAND PRESSURE POINTS

concert. The first points, used to stimulate the adrenal glands, are located two and one–half inches above and one inch to either side of the navel. Hold your hands with the palms across the abdomen, with the fingertips pointing toward each other. Now using a circular motion, massage with the fingertips of each hand deep into the abdomen in this area, just below the rib cage. Do not massage these points too close to bedtime, as you may not be able to go to sleep.

The second set of points which stimulates the brain, is located on each side of the chest, running from a point on the collarbone directly below the ears vertically down to the armpit. Use your thumbs or fingers to massage with firm pressure in a circular motion all the way down this line. These points may feel rather sensitive or painful at first, but as the massaging takes effect, the tenderness will decrease, and you will become more alert.

SLEEPLESSNESS OR EMOTIONAL UPSET
Place the tips of the four fingers of each hand over the frontal eminence on each side of the forehead. This is the slight bulge on either side of the forehead, between the eyebrows and the hairline. Feel for a faint pulse in this area, and hold with gentle fingertip pressure on these points for two to five minutes. Usually, within a few minutes you will begin to feel relaxed enough to sleep, or your troubling thoughts will begin to melt away. Pressing these points helps to normalize the adrenal glands after an upsetting event.

Another point for sedating the adrenal glands is located on the posterior fontanel on the top rear of

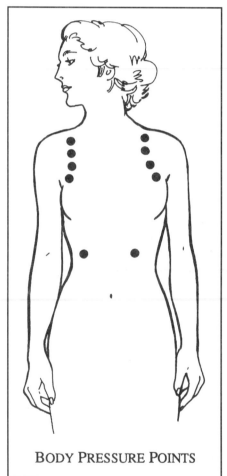

BODY PRESSURE POINTS

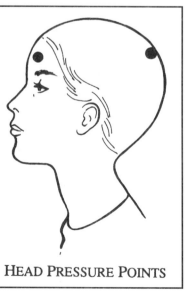

HEAD PRESSURE POINTS

the head—the "soft spot" on the back of a baby's head. Feel for the slight pulse, and hold for two to ten minutes, to calm upset or ease yourself into sleep.

Warm Soak and Stroke

A wonderful way to relax before bedtime is to do a self-massage in your bath. You can use these self-massage techniques anywhere, at any time during the day, to work on easily reached trouble spots that accumulate tension.

Be sure that your bathroom is nice and warm when you begin. Add one pound of Epsom salts and leftover Rejuvelac to a warm (not hot) bath. Periodically add a little hot water if necessary to maintain the temperature for twenty to thirty minutes. The Epsom salts promote the eliminative activity of the skin, carrying through the work of elimination begun by stimulating the circulation of blood and lymph with massage. You do not need to use oil for this massage, since the bath water will provide lubrication.

Sitting up in the tub, begin with the neck. Using the thumb and fingers, grasp the muscle on either side of the spine at the back of the neck. Move gradually up and down each side of the spine, pinching and releasing the muscle, going down as far as you can and up to the base of the skull. Concentrate on the areas that feel tight and sore. Bend your neck back and hang your head forward as you continue to pinch and knead the muscles. Do some neck rolls to the sides to loosen up the neck, then massage the neck muscles some more.

From the neck, move out toward the shoulders. Rest the heels of the hands on the tops of the shoulders against the neck, with the fingers curled over the back of the shoulders. Now, slide your hands forward with a firm, smooth, sliding pressure, so that your elbows come down over the chest. Repeat this sliding movement, gradually working out from the neck to the shoulder, pressing as hard as you wish. Feel the heat in your skin as you slide your hands firmly over the muscles.

Now, work on one shoulder at a time with the opposite hand, squeezing all around the shoulder joint. Begin with gentle squeezing, then increase until you are squeezing as hard as is comfortable.

Next, work on the arms, always moving toward the heart. Work on one hand and arm, and then switch to the other. Begin by massaging each finger from the tip up to the palm. Take the time to squeeze, stroke, and shake each of the fingers and the thumb, working the blood and lymph back toward the heart. Now, squeeze and massage the hands, stroking firmly along the bones, always moving toward the heart to flush out the wastes and stagnant blood. Work your way up the arm, kneading and squeezing the muscles. Work around the elbow, massaging any tender spots you find, and moving up toward the armpits. Finish with strong upward strokes, using the whole opposite hand, with the fingers wrapped around the arm, to push the blood and lymph back toward the heart. If you feel tender spots, you may be encountering areas of congested lymph. Work on them, and then move everything onward, squeezing and stroking toward the heart. Take the time to do some shoulder rolls to loosen up your shoulders as you work.

Next, massage your legs. Use both hands to work on one foot and calf, then go on to the other. Bend one knee so that you can rest the foot on the opposite thigh. Squeeze and massage the toes from the tip toward the foot, to force the blood back toward the heart. Slide your index finger back and forth between the toes, feeling the wonderful relaxation spreading through your body. Grasp all your toes with one hand, and with the other hand bend the foot back and forth. Massage along the bones on the top of the foot, and knead deeply into the sole, gently moving up toward the leg.

Keeping your knee bent with the foot resting on the opposite thigh, massage the calf, kneading and squeezing. Then use strong, firm strokes with both hands to move the circulation up the calf into the thighs. When you have finished one calf, work on the other foot and calf.

Now, straighten the legs in front of you to work on the knees and thighs. Work on one knee at a time, squeezing and kneading with both hands behind and around the sides of the knee. Next, grasp the top of one thigh between thumb and fingers, squeeze, and let the muscle slip out of your hand. Work your way all over the thighs in this manner to stimulate the circulation. Then stroke strongly up the thigh with both hands curved around the leg. Finish by stroking the insides of both thighs, up toward the groin. Remember that massaging toward the heart helps to flush the veins, promoting circulation and cleansing.

After your massage, get out of the bath and dry briskly with a coarse towel. Wrap in a robe or towel and get into bed and relax for fifteen minutes, or prepare for sleep. The cleansing properties of the Epsom salts, activated by the self–massage, will continue to draw wastes out of your skin through the night.

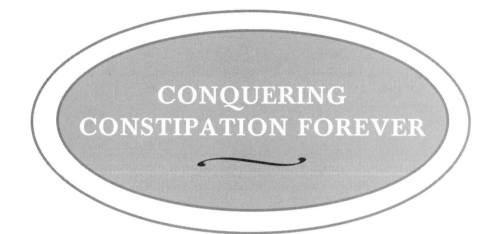

CONQUERING CONSTIPATION FOREVER

*R*ejuvenation truly begins within. The key to youthful beauty is a properly functioning digestive system—an "inner spa" that functions around the clock, absorbing the nutrients needed to build fresh new cells and cleansing your body of toxic wastes that age your appearance and drain your energy.

Digestion begins in the mouth, where the teeth grind the food and saliva is released by the salivary glands. The enzyme ptyalin in saliva begins to break down the starches, converting them to sugars, and some nutrients are absorbed right in the mouth. When the food is swallowed, it travels down the esophagus, moved along by wavelike muscular contractions known as peristalsis. The food enters the stomach, where hydrochloric acid and digestive enzymes break it down into particles to be assimilated. The resultant nutrients are absorbed through the stomach wall.

The food now moves into the duodenum, which is the beginning of more than twenty feet of small intestine. Several small ducts empty into the duodenum. One comes from the gallbladder, a small sac that stores a liver secretion called bile, which helps to digest fats. Another duct deposits juices from the pancreas that are rich in enzymes that break down partially digested proteins.

After food leaves the duodenum, most of the nutrients are absorbed in the small intestine, through tiny finger like projections called villi. These nutrients are carried by the bloodstream and the lymph to the liver to be purified before they are distributed to the cells of the body. Material that is not absorbed while it is in the small intestine is waste, and it passes into the colon. In a healthy colon, this waste is excreted as feces in six to twelve hours.

I am convinced, based on my observations of many clients, that undigested starches and proteins are really the root of much illness and premature aging. If we learn to eat properly so that our food is properly assimilated and eliminated, many symptoms of toxicity will be prevented, and the aging process will be slowed. Bad breath, unpleasant body odor, bags under the eyes, low–back pain, obesity, cellulite—all these are symptoms produced by undigested, decomposing food in the intestine.

Dairy products and other foods that produce mucoid deposits line the intestinal walls, preventing the proper absorption of nutrients. Many people overeat simply because the nutrients in their food are not being absorbed through their mucus–coated intestinal walls. They feel hungry and eat more and more because they are starving for vital vitamins and minerals; but only the calories are readily absorbed, and so they gain weight. Eating simple, easily digestible foods in proper combinations helps to prevent the buildup of mucous deposits so that nutrients are properly absorbed and cravings are eliminated.

Place your finger on your abdomen on the pelvic bone just above your right thigh, and trace a vertical line up to just above the level of your navel. Continue across to your left side, and trace another vertical line down to the same abdominal point above your left thigh. Your finger has traced the approximate route of your colon, some five to six feet from beginning to end, including its curves and folds. (This is the area where many people mistakenly say they have a "stomach ache.")

When the mixture of food and digestive juices, known as chyme, leaves the small intestine and enters the colon, it is in a semi–liquid state. The first part of the colon, in the lower right abdomen, is known as the cecum. The chyme is pushed by peristaltic action from the cecum, past the area of the appendix, and up along the right side of the abdomen. As it moves along, moisture is absorbed through the colon wall into the lymphatic system, to become blood plasma. The colon makes its turn just under the right rib cage in the area of the liver and gallbladder, and the now mushy food moves across the abdomen above the navel, turning again just below the left rib cage in the area of the spleen and pancreas. By this time, the stool has become more solid, and as it moves downward toward the floor of the pelvis, it exerts a pressure that finally triggers the muscles to evacuate the contents.

Unfortunately, what I have described is only an ideal digestive scenario. For many people, the waste moves through the colon much too slowly, leading to constipation and irregular elimination. Once the stool gets slowed down, the colon is no longer able to exert its normal peristaltic action, its nerve signals shut down, and hard, dehydrated waste begins to lodge in pockets in the colon and to get plastered on the intestinal wall. This stagnant waste contains many toxic substances, which are gradually reabsorbed by the blood into the system, creating what is known as toxemia or toxicity.

Because of mild body toxicity, I observe a wide range of symptoms in my

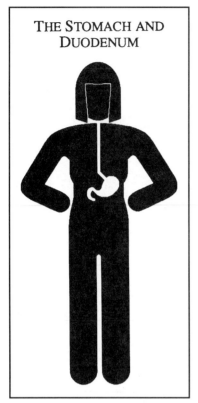

THE STOMACH AND DUODENUM

clients who are constipated—fatigue, flatulence, headaches, irritability, nausea, nervousness, depression, protruding abdomen due to bloating, and obesity. They often have coated tongues, bad breath, body odors, dark circles under the eyes, and brittle hair and nails. While some medical authorities in the United States might disagree with this long list of symptoms, a group of England's most eminent physicians, at a meeting of the Royal Society of Medicine, presented an amazingly long list of ailments, affecting virtually every part of the body, that are caused either directly or indirectly by toxemia arising from malfunctions of the bowels.

Many factors can contribute to the slowing of bowel transit time and constipation, including improper diet, inadequate water consumption, failure to respond to the urge to eliminate, emotional stress, lack of exercise, and the use of painkillers and other medications. Regular toning exercises, such as the Digestion Toning Postures on page 128, help to keep the abdominal organs functioning at their peak, assuring that your "inner spa" will be cleansing and rejuvenating your whole body.

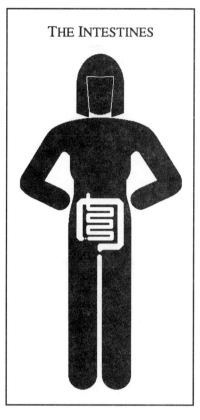

THE INTESTINES

CONSTIPATION AND AGING

Many people think their bowels are moving normally, and yet they may actually be constipated. If you must often strain to move your bowels, or have a bloated, uncomfortable abdomen, you have symptoms of constipation. Populations who eat healthy diets of clean, whole, natural foods high in fiber do not suffer from such symptoms, and their stools are full, large, and soft.

Ideally, elimination of feces should occur in direct proportion to the amount of food eaten. This means that if you eat three meals each day, you should have three bowel movements each day. It makes sense that your colon would promptly eliminate the waste from what you eat. Of coarse, this goal cannot be reached overnight by people who have had long–standing problems with constipation. As you follow my suggestions on the 21–Day Program, you should find your own elimination pattern moving toward this ideal.

What happens in your colon can affect every part of your body. Putrefying waste trapped in the colon produces a number of toxic substances, some of which have been implicated as causes of cancer. These substances pass through the colon wall and enter the bloodstream and lymph, where they are carried throughout the body. These poisons can produce symptoms in the nervous system such as headaches, depression, mental dullness, or a case of the blahs. The liver and the colon are directly connected by their blood supply. It is the liver's job to remove the toxic substances from the body by filtering impurities out of the blood. The liver can become overtaxed and damaged by all the extra toxins from the colon. Toxic and incompletely digested waste can also impair the function of the kidneys, whose job it is to filter waste from the blood before excreting excess water. A high–protein diet also places a heavy burden on the kidneys.

The skin is another organ of elimination that can be over–stressed by a constipated colon. Not only can the complexion develop wrinkles and eruptions, or become sallow or blotchy as a direct result of toxic substances accumulating in the skin, but offensive body odor is also a reflection of a congested, unclean colon. Similarly, bad breath is often a sign that there is a toxic condition in the intestines. When the putrefying waste makes its way through the bloodstream to the lungs, it fouls the breath.

Constipation may also increase the risk for breast disease, including lumpy and cystic breasts and breast cancer. According to a 1981 report in Lancet, the British medical journal, a study of fifteen hundred women at a California breast clinic showed that breast diseases were relatively rare among women who had bowel movements at least once a day, while women who had two or fewer bowel movements a week had more than four times greater incidence of breast problems. More recently, the American Journal of Public Health reported in January 1989 that a study of seven thousand women showed a slightly increased incidence of breast cancer among women who reported constipation problems, as indicated by infrequent bowel movements or hard stools. The explanation may lie partly in the changes in intestinal flora that occur with constipation. The friendly bacteria in an unconstipated colon help detoxify bile salts and excess estrogen, which have been implicated in the development of breast lumps and cancer.

Poisons from the colon can weaken and stress the heart, cause pain and stiffness in the joints, weaken and fatigue the muscles, rob you of your beauty and your health, and age you prematurely. And it is not just the poisonous substances being reabsorbed into the bloodstream that cause problems, but a constipated colon can also bulge and press on the neighboring organs, further impairing the function of the liver, the heart, the reproductive organs, and the kidneys.

Constipation also affects the bacteria in your colon. Your intestinal tract has two very different types of bacteria. The so-called coliform bacteria are the ones that cause putrefaction, producing toxic substances. These putrefactive bacteria thrive in the oxygen-starved, alkaline environment produced by an improper diet and a constipated colon. The beneficial bacteria are Lactobacillus bacteria, primarily Lactobacillus acidophilus and L. Bifidus. These "friendly" bacteria, which require an oxygenated, acid environment, manufacture B vitamins and vitamin K in the intestine, and produce digestive enzymes.

A healthy colon should contain at least 85 percent beneficial bacillus, and no more than 15 percent of the coliform "bad guys." But most people in our society show a reversed ratio of 85 percent coliform and fifteen percent bacillus. As you cleanse your colon I want you to realize you are restoring the proper balance of good bacteria. While it is possible to buy Lactobacillus supplements in a health-food store, I recommend that you promote the good bacteria in your intestines by drinking Rejuvelac on page 88. Rejuvelac is full of Lactobacillus species and other friendly bacteria. It contains natural lactic acid, which helps to destroy the harmful bacteria, and enzymes that help digestion. It is no wonder that Rejuvelac has earned a reputation for promoting a beautiful complexion. Clear, youthful skin is simply a reflection of a clean, healthy colon.

COLON CLEANSING

A great deal of the waste that you want to remove from your body during the cleansing program will end up in the colon–not only the residue from your food, but also toxic waste that has been delivered into the colon by the lymph system. Your body cannot be completely clean as long as your colon is blocked, so it is essential during any cleansing program to remove all the debris from the colon. I also consider colon cleansing an essential part of any truly effective weight–loss program, since it helps to remove toxins from the body that might otherwise end up being stored in the excess fat cells.

Laxatives are not sufficient for cleaning the colon; in fact, laxatives dehydrate the body, and often leave old layers of dried feces on the colon wall, allowing only more recent waste to push through and evacuate. Even though the bowels are being evacuated, a condition of constipation exists, causing degeneration of the nerves and muscles of the colon, so that even more laxatives are needed.

COLON HYDROTHERAPY

A much better way to cleanse the colon is to flush it with clean, purified water. Colon hydrotherapy was first recorded in 1500 B.C. in the Ebers Papyrus. In the fourth and fifth centuries B.C., Hippocrates reported using enemas for treating fevers, and the Essenes used water therapy to rid the colon of uncleanliness and the body of disease. In modern times, colonic irrigation was quite popular among some physicians in the 1920's, 1930's, and 1940's, and then it fell out of favor. Now, with safe, effective, and sterile equipment, colonic irrigation is once again being recognized as a valuable adjunct to health care.

Colonic irrigation is a gentle warm–water washing of the colon that cleanses the entire length from the rectum all the way up to the cecum at the beginning of the colon. To receive a colonic, you lie on your side and the colon hygienist inserts a small disposable tube in the anus. At the foot of the table, a hygienic colonic irrigation machine regulates the water pressure, temperature, and volume. After insertion, as you relax on your back, the water is slowly and gently infused into your colon. Before any excessive pressure is felt, the direction of water flow is reversed, and the contents of the colon are evacuated through the tube. The most important thing for you to do during this process is to relax.

Most people are amazed at how much mucus, feces, and excess gas is removed from their colon during their first colonic. And after expressing their initial skepticism, most people find a colonic to be a very pleasant, relaxing experience.

You may wonder whether you will become dependent on colonics, but actually the opposite is true. When colonics are done properly, with a low–pressure technique, they exercise and tone the muscles of the colon, improving its peristaltic activity. Generally, one colonic is not enough to completely empty the colon. At the Inner Beauty Institute, we usually recommend that our clients begin with four to six sessions over about a three–week period. Clients who choose to go on to do a deeper cleansing after that may require many more sessions, depending on their health history, age, and personal objectives.

You may have heard that a colonic will wash away the beneficial bacteria in the colon. On the contrary, if your colon has been constipated for some time, it is really helpful to flush away the putrefactive bacteria that have accumulated there. A colon–cleansing program, along with a proper diet, will help to change the environment in the colon to make it more hospitable to the beneficial lactobacillus bacteria. Colon therapists generally recommend supplementary bacteria for nutritional support while the colon is getting back into proper balance.

Colonic irrigations not only clean the colon, but they also produce a feeling of well–being. We tend to have a lot of negative mental programming about our eliminative systems, and in fact the taboos about elimination often contribute to constipation problems. Colonic irrigations can help to create a new awareness of how it feels to release and let go of the waste that has been trapped in your body. After a series of colonic irrigations, you may also feel an increased energy level, your skin will be radiant, your eyes clear, and your digestion will be better than ever.

People bothered by protruding abdomens and excess weight find immediate relief with a colonic. During a cleansing program, they often eliminate as much as five to fifteen pounds just from cleaning out their intestines, and when the accumulated gas is removed along with the excess feces, their tummies become flat.

One of the most rewarding parts of my work is seeing the truly miraculous changes that occur after clients have had colonic irrigations. One of my clients, named Marlene, is the owner of a travel agency. She does a great deal of traveling in the course of her business, and a combination of restaurant and airline food, jet lag, and stress had caused her to develop a severe constipation problem over the years. Even before she came to me for help, she had known that her body was toxic. Marlene had begun to clean up her diet, and she was making an effort to get more sleep and regular exercise. Even though she had improved her lifestyle, it had not really helped her constipation problem. She still was not eliminating more than a couple of times a week. As a result, her system was very toxic. She had terrible headaches, and dreaded her menstrual periods because they were so uncomfortable. Her skin was very blotchy, and she felt generally sluggish.

Marlene heard about my clinic in Sausalito from friends in the airline industry who were my clients, and finally she came to see me in desperation. After consulting our physician, she began her cleansing program with a series of colonics. After about three months, Marlene's skin was really beginning to clear, its texture had improved, and she had developed a healthy glow. Her headaches had also gone away, and her periods were becoming much more comfortable. For someone else with similar symptoms, who had not already made an effort to improve her diet, it might have taken much longer to eliminate the symptoms of toxicity. In Marlene's case, the colonics made all the difference in turning things around and changing her whole outlook on life.

How to Select a Colon Therapist

I have suggested that you have at least three colonic irrigations during your 21–Day Cleansing and Rejuvenation Program. Ideally, all of these cleansings should be performed by a professional colon hygienist. Three professional colonic irrigations may cost more money than you can afford at this time, or you may not be able to locate a colon hygienist in your area, so I have also provided instructions for giving yourself a cleansing enema at home. If it is at all possible, however, please arrange for a least one colonic irrigation with a professional, since this will be a much more effective cleansing treatment than an enema. Preferably, if you can have only one professional colonic, schedule it ahead of time for Day 15.

As always, the best source of information about a colon hygienist is through personal referrals. Ask your friends if they can recommend a colon hygienist in your area. If not, consult the International Association of Colon Therapy at (916) 222–1498. If no one is listed in your area, look in the yellow pages of your telephone directory under Colonic Irrigation. In some states, you will not find this listing. In that case, look under Naturopaths, Chiropractors, Holistic Health Care, or Health Spas–these practitioners and facilities may be able to refer you to a colon therapist. You can also ask for referrals at your local health–food store, or look in the classified section of an alternative newspaper such as Common Ground. You might also call a local hospital and ask to speak with a nurse on duty; at least one nurse will probably know of colonic irrigation facilities in the area.

Once you have the name of a colon therapist, you are ready to phone and ask questions to determine whether this person is the right professional for you. Here are some questions to ask and points to cover in the conversation.

1. Ask if the colon hygienist uses modern equipment, as opposed to the older gravity–style equipment, which is harder to sterilize. The newer kind of equipment is characterized by separate inflow and outflow water systems and, when entering the colon, uses low water pressure.

2. Ask whether the hygienist uses disposable tubing and speculum. Disposable equipment has become the standard for the modern practice of colon therapy. If the therapist does not use disposable equipment and is the only person available, ask how the tubing is sterilized. The only acceptable method is autoclaving.

3. Ask if the hygienist uses filtered water for the colonic irrigation. This has become a standard of good practice.

4. Ask the hygienist if he or she provides nutritional counseling in the session. Prevention of future constipation problems is one of the primary objectives of colon hygiene, and proper diet is the key.

5. Ask if the hygienist is familiar with the use of abdominal massage during the colonic. Massage helps to release trapped material from the colon.

6. Ask whether the therapist offers an herbal steam in addition to the colonic irrigation. Many do not, but if you find someone who does offer it, be sure to take advantage of it; it really enhances the cleansing process.

If a colonic irrigation is a completely new experience for you, it is important that the hygienist put you at ease about the procedure. But no matter how pleasant the therapist sounds on the phone, look elsewhere if he or she is not using modern, disposable or properly sterilized equipment.

While having your colonic, use the breathing techniques and affirmations you have already learned during this program. Take nice deep breaths into the abdomen, especially if you feel any cramping. Practicing deep–breathing techniques will help you to achieve a deeper release. If you feel a little apprehensive because this is your first colonic, or because you are not accustomed to having a stranger touch that part of your body, use your affirmations and breathing to calm and center yourself. Do not be afraid to discuss your feelings with the therapist; it is part of the colon hygienist's job to help you to relax and to allay your anxieties.

Hot Castor–Oil Abdominal Wrap

A perfect way to end your cleansing fast on Day 14 and to prepare for a colonic irrigation is to use a Hot Castor–Oil Abdominal Wrap. This abdominal wrap has the same benefits as expensive herbal wraps in salon, but its effects are more lasting. The Hot Castor–Oil Wrap helps to break down the toxins stored in the tissues, and to loosen the waste in the colon so that it can be flushed away. The wrap also helps to detoxify the lymph system, since the major lymph drainage goes into the colon. At the Inner Beauty Institute, we have observed that the results of colon cleansing are enhanced when a Hot Castor–Oil Wrap is used the night before.

This Castor–Oil Wrap was popularized by the renowned psychic Edgar Cayce, who recommended it in thousands of his health readings. Many health practitioners, including myself, follow some of Cayce's recommendations. This wrap is useful for a wide variety of problems, including headaches, abdominal tenderness, problems with the digestive system and the sex organs, menstrual cramps, and muscular tension. In addition, the Hot Castor–Oil Wrap has a particularly relaxing effect on the nervous system.

To make your own Hot Castor–Oil Abdominal Wrap you will need the following materials:

> 4 ounces of Castor Oil
> Bowl or pan
> Piece of large, soft wool flanne
>   (16 inches by 12 to 18 inches)
> Electric heating pad
> Large plastic bag (such as a garbage bag or dry
>   cleaner's bag)
> Large towel to lie on

Pour some of the castor oil into the bowl or pan and soak the flannel cloth in the oil. Then wring it out thoroughly, so that the cloth is just moist; it should not be dripping wet. Now, fold the cloth in half so that it measures eight inches in one dimension. It will reach from the groin up to just under the breasts. The long side, twelve to eighteen inches, will reach all the way across the abdomen. Place a towel on your bed to avoid soiling. Plug in the heating pad by your bedside.

Lie down and place the folded cloth over your abdomen, then place the plastic bag over the cloth, and tuck it underneath you. Finally, position the heating pad over the entire arrangement and set it to medium heat.

Enjoy the wonderfully soothing benefits of the abdominal wrap for at least one and one–half hours, or even up to two to three hours if you wish. Relax, watch TV, read, do some gentle breathing exercises, or just do nothing. Some people simply fall asleep because the Castor–Oil Wrap is so calming.

While this wrap is designed to be used over the front of the abdomen, you can apply it to other parts of your body as well. For example, if you are having low–back problems or kidney problems, it is fine to use it on your back.

When you are finished using the Hot Castor–Oil Abdominal Wrap, place the moist flannel cloth in a plastic bag and keep it in your refrigerator. You can use it over and over, as many times as you wish.

Remove the castor oil from your skin by taking a bath with two tablespoons of baking soda dissolved in it, or simply let the castor oil continue to soak in overnight for extra moisturizing benefits.

No one really knows exactly why this Castor–Oil Wrap works. The oil from the castor bean has long been a popular folk remedy. It has been applied externally for all sorts of skin problems, rubbed on the breasts to increase the flow of milk, and rubbed into the chest to relieve chest cold or bronchitis. It is also used as a base in lipstick and other makeup, because it is so stable and soothing to the skin.

Although I am recommending the Hot Castor–Oil Wrap specifically for the purpose of cleansing, it also has a tremendously calming effect on the central nervous system, helping people to fall asleep with ease. It is also a fantastic remedy for menstrual cramps, constipation, indigestion and many other abdominal discomforts. Feel free to use it whenever you wish.

Tummy Massage

Become familiar with this Tummy Massage before attempting to give yourself an enema. A colon therapist will administer a similar massage when you receive your professional colonic irrigation. When used along with colon cleansing, this Tummy Massage helps to loosen deposits in the colon and to gently work the waste down toward the rectum to be eliminated.

Lie on your back on a firm surface with your knees up, to relax the colon and abdominal organs. Warm a little castor oil in your hands and start on the lower right side of your abdomen, massaging with your fingers in a circular motion. Press as deeply as is comfortable. As you massage deeply, you may encounter areas that are tender. Do not be alarmed by this; just make note of the tender places. Breathe into them and massage them away.

Continue to work your way up the right side to just below the rib cage, then move across the upper abdomen above the navel, massaging deeply in firm circular motions, again noting any tender areas. You may feel some hard masses as you move across the abdomen. This may be congestion in your colon. Move across the tummy to your left side. Work slowly, trying to relax into any area that feels tender. These tender areas provide you with feedback on where your colon may be congested.

Now, work your way down along the left side of your abdomen. Massage deeply, all the way down to the pelvic bone on the left. You have now massaged all along the course of the colon, following the natural direction in which the waste moves out of your body.

Once you have gone around the colon, go up again under the rib cage on the right. This area is the home of your liver. Massage there and feel if there is any hardness or tenderness. Then massage below the rib cage in the middle of the abdomen. Press in under the rib cage; this is the solar plexus, where the diaphragm is located. We often hold a lot of tension and stress in this area. If anything feels tender or tight, breathe into it to loosen it up and really relax. As you massage, you will feel a release of tension. Massage under the left side of the rib cage, in the area of the spleen, breathing and relaxing into any tender spots.

Allow fifteen or twenty minutes for your Tummy Massage, ending with palming of the abdomen. Generate heat in your hands by rubbing your palms together for at least 30 seconds, and then lay your hands on your abdomen in any area that feels tight, or where you feel you want to direct healing, loving energy. Allow the warmth to go into your tummy, into all your abdominal organs, helping them to let go of the waste, congestion, and tension.

How to Give Yourself a Cleansing Enema

In our culture, we do not grow up associating colon cleansing with regular health maintenance. Yet many of the great natural–healing clinics insist that clients on fasting programs take one or two enemas every day to facilitate the detoxification process. I realize that many people still cling to the old destructive taboos and fears about this part of their body. If you do have inhibitions, try to break through and allow yourself to do colon cleansing during this program. The overall benefits will be greatly enhanced.

If for some reason you are not able to obtain colonic irrigations, you can give yourself a gentle cleansing enema at home instead. You can also have both colonics and enemas. Enemas are not able to flush the entire colon as effectively as a colonic, but they can still be very helpful. Do not hesitate to give yourself an enema every day that you happen to be troubled by cleansing reactions. The enema will really help to clear up any uncomfortable symptoms.

To give yourself an enema, use any standard enema bag from the drugstore. Also buy some petroleum jelly or lubricating jelly.

I recommend that you give yourself the enema lying on your slant board, since lying in the head–down antigravity position helps the water to travel further into the colon. You can also lie on the floor, or in your bathtub–wherever is more comfortable for you. Prepare the area where you will be doing the enema by arranging a towel to lie on. Find a place where you can hang the bag so that the bottom of the bag is about one or two feet above your rectum. It is very important not to hang the bag too high, because you want the water to trickle in slowly and gently.

Fill the enema bag with warm purified water. Add a couple of drops of fresh lemon juice to help break up fecal impactions. Be careful not to get any seeds in the bag. Unclamp the tube and let a little water run out of the enema nozzle to remove air from the tubing. Then clamp the tube shut, hang the enema bag, and lie on your back with your knees up. Apply a small amount of petroleum jelly or lubricating jelly to the tip of the enema tube and gently insert the tip into your rectum. Release the clamp and let the water trickle in slowly, as much as you can comfortably hold. This first fill will be going into the lower portion of the colon, on the left side of the abdomen. Let the water run in until you just begin to sense discomfort–perhaps pressure at the rectum, or a general feeling of fullness. Stop at this point, clamp the tube, and go to the toilet. If you are able, hold the water in for a moment, and massage your abdomen gently on the lower left side to work the water up into the colon and loosen the material before you go to the toilet.

After you have evacuated your bowel, return to the enema setup and lie on your left side. Once again let the water gently trickle in so that you stop just before you sense discomfort or urgency. This time hold the water in if you can. Massage from the lower right abdomen up the right side, across the top of the abdomen, and down the left side, as you did when you practiced your Tummy Massage. You will be loosening the waste and working it out of your colon. Evacuate again, and then fill your colon one more time, this time lying on the right side. Let the water run slowly in, as much as you can hold. You will feel the water gurgling around. You want it to go as far in as it can, down into the right side of the colon. Massage once again up the right side, across the top of the abdomen, and down the left side, to break up pockets of hardened waste.

On the second and subsequent fills with the enema, use as much water as you comfortably can, and then allow your bowels to completely empty themselves. With each successive evacuation, you will be able to hold more water in your colon, since more space will be emptied out. The more water you can get into your colon, the more effective the enema will be.

You may find it somewhat awkward to lie on your side on the slant board. However, as you become more familiar with the entire enema procedure, you will be able to move around a little more easily and do more massaging.

After your enema, you may feel quite sleepy, or your may feel surprisingly invigorated. Allow time after your enema to relax quietly, and do not get too far away from the toilet, because you may still feel the urge to evacuate your bowels

Colon cleansing is the key to completely cleaning out your body. As you practice effective and safe cleansing of your systems of elimination, you will become more sensitive to the miraculous workings of your body. Just as you have released the waste from your cells, tissues, and organs, you have also released negative emotional and mental patterns. The cleansing process brings body, mind, emotions, and spirit into greater harmony. By the end of your Cleansing and Rejuvenation Program, you will be lighter, clearer, and wonderfully rejuvenated.

CONQUERING CONSTIPATION FOREVER

We have examined what happens when waste is not promptly eliminated from the colon and its poisonous contents are allowed to reenter the bloodstream, causing symptoms throughout the body. I truly believe that this internal pollution underlies a great deal of illness. Overweight, lethargy, headache, poor skin condition, unpleasant body odor, low–back pain, premature aging–all the symptoms listed in the Toxicity Symptom Checklist on page 22–can result from constipation. These symptoms are early warning signs of more serious problems that can develop if the constipation is not corrected. As you go through the 21–Day Program and beyond, please repeat the Toxicity Symptom Checklist to see what improvements have occurred now that you have begun to incorporate into your life techniques to reduce toxicity and end constipation once and for all.

It was the British physician Denis Burkitt who first called widespread attention to the relationship between diet, constipation, and disease. Burkitt was one of a number of British doctors working with native villagers in Africa. He noticed a striking difference between the elimination habits of the natives and those of the Englishmen. The Africans' meals would pass through their digestive tracts to be eliminated in about twenty–four hours, whereas for the English it generally took three days, and sometimes as long as two weeks. Not only did the Africans eliminate their waste much more rapidly, but their stools were also large and soft, in sharp contrast to the generally small, hard, difficult–to–pass stools of the British doctors. The Africans were eating unprocessed natural foods high in fiber, whereas the Englishmen were eating the typical "civilized" diet high in refined white flour, sugar, and saturated fats. Not only were the Africans free of constipation, but they were also free of many of the diseases that have become plagues of modern civilization, such as heart disease, colon and rectal cancer, appendicitis, hemorrhoids, obesity, and varicose veins. As a result of Burkitt's observations, fiber became a popular supplement in modern Western diets.

I have gone into graphic detail to help you consider the question of whether you have a problem with constipation. Are your stools soft and full, or are they small and hard? A constipated system is one where waste moves through the bowel slowly, and its hard consistency causes strain and eventual damage to your body. Even when your bowel movements seem to be regular and normal, they may be squeezing their way past an accumulation of hardened, dried waste somewhere in the colon.

Moreover, remember that the waste should move through your system to be eliminated promptly after it has been digested. You may think you are doing fine if you have one bowel movement each day, but if you eat three meals a day, that means there are two other meals backed up in your colon, waiting to be eliminated. As you heal and cleanse your digestive system and colon, you will begin to move toward the ideal of one bowel movement per day for each meal eaten each day. It is a natural, common–sense relationship between what goes in and what comes out.

Earlier in this chapter, I taught you how to do a Tummy Massage that follows the course of your colon, feeling deep inside your abdomen for areas that seem hard or sore. Now that you know where your colon is located, you may begin to realize that your protruding tummy, or your frequent abdominal pains, may be caused by a constipated colon. Many people think they have a stomach ache, when the problem is not in their stomach at all.

The story of one of my clients, Doreen, illustrates this point very dramatically. Doreen and her husband have their own business, and she also spends a great deal of time caring for a disabled son. From morning to night, Doreen is on the run, taking care of her business and taking care of her family. She is one of those people who had never thought of herself as constipated, even though she would have bowel movements only every second or third day. That was the way it had been for her mother, and she though it was just normal for her.

Over a couple of years' time, Doreen had had more or less constant pain in her upper abdomen, in the area near the liver. She had been to many different doctors, and most recently had had gallbladder studies. The doctors were very concerned because they could find no explanation for the pain, and had recommended exploratory surgery. Fortunately for Doreen, her massage therapist noticed congestion in her abdominal area and sent her to the Inner Beauty Institute. We found that she had severely impacted waste in her colon that had become so hard it was impossible to dislodge with regular bowel movements. After three colonic irrigation treatments, Doreen's pain went away, and the only time it comes back now is when she becomes constipated. She has learned to know her body well enough to recognize what is causing the pain when it occurs, and what foods may have caused the constipation. As an added benefit, Doreen began to experience a much more satisfying sex life with the use of deep breathing, as she learned to release not just the waste from her bowels but also the tension from her pelvic area.

Because the focus of the entire 21–Day Program is on cleansing the systems of elimination, just about everything you have learned so far will help in your battle against constipation. To begin with, be sure to drink at least eight glasses of pure, clean water each day. This fluid intake may be in the form of plain purified water or the sweetened Hydrating Drink, herbal teas, Oxygenation Cocktail, or other beverages recommended in this program. These healthful, toxin–free drinks ensure that your colon is properly hydrated, bathing and cleansing your cells, tissues, and organs of elimination. A correctly combined diet of fresh, natural foods, including plenty of raw fruits and vegetables and fresh juices, provides water content and minerals for proper bowel function, as well as the fiber to move the waste through your intestines quickly and cleanly.

Some foods are very dehydrating and thus can lead to constipation. A particularly insidious culprit is bread. All the people I have ever worked with on constipation problems have improved when they eliminated bread from their diet. People who are constipated should not eat bread, with the possible exception of dark pumpernickel made without yeast, such as Ruhrtaler pumpernickel, available in many health–food and specialty gourmet stores. Also, avoid mucoid forming foods such as cheese, since they tend to coat the intestinal wall and impair absorption. Hard cheese is as difficult to digest as bread. It absorbs moisture out of the system and produces dehydration. I realize that many people will have a hard time giving up cheese entirely; my advice is to consider it a special treat rather than an everyday staple.

Help your digestive system by adding friendly bacteria in the form of

ANTI-CONSTIPATION DIET

Look over this table of good foods and bad foods for fighting constipation. How many of the Foods to Avoid have been staples in your regular diet?

FOODS TO EAT

Fresh fruits and vegetables, including raw ones and fresh-squeezed juices
Prunes and prune juice
Whole grains—one serving per day
Sprouts
Fibrous foods in general
Lots of steamed vegetables when you eat protein
Potassium-rich foods, such as vegetables and Potassium Broth
At least eight glasses of water—in the form of Hydrating Drink, purified water, herb teas, broth, and other fluids
Cold-pressed vegetable oils, such as olive, sesame, and safflower—two tablespoons per day
Fermented foods, such as Rejuvelac and sauerkraut
Hot Lemon-Water Flush
Supplements, such as aloe vera juice, liquid minerals, Lactobacillus supplement, and intestinal cleanser

FOODS TO AVOID

Bread
Cheese
Salt
Refined sugar
White flour
Candies, cookies, and pastries
Excessive coffee and black tea
Carbonated beverages/Alcoholic beverages
Processed foods—canned, salted foods
Salted snack foods
Fried foods
Excessive animal protein
Very hot or very cold foods

Rejuvelac on page 88 or a Lactobacillus supplement, and use digestive enzymes if you combine meals improperly or eat a lot of protein. I describe digestive enzymes on page 74. Proper eating habits are essential for eliminating constipation. Always eat slowly and calmly, be sure to chew your food well, and avoid overeating. Adequate exercise, such as walking, swimming, or trampolining, helps to keep your bowel function regular, as do slant–board exercises. Yoga exercises, such as the Yoga Arch Pose Variations on page 124 and the Digestion Toning Postures on page 128, help to promote proper digestion and elimination. Sitz baths, especially the cold "Youth Bath" I described on page 154, bring vastly increased circulation to the abdominal organs, and can be very helpful in aiding digestion, expelling gas, and encouraging proper bowel function.

Regardless of your busy schedule, always heed nature's call. Repressing the urge to move your bowels when you have to go is one of the most common contributing factors in chronic constipation. Based on extensive research with my clients, I have concluded that constipation problems can often be traced back to early childhood embarrassment about going to the bathroom, or to having to "hold it" when it was necessary to wait to use the toilet. This early conditioning can still be undone in adulthood. Establish the habit of trying to have a bowel movement first thing every morning, whether you feel the urge or not. Be prepared to take fifteen minutes if necessary, do not strain, and just be patient. If you bowels are weak, they will take longer to respond. Try breathing deeply and bending forward, and elevate your feet on a low stool if necessary. Also try using the colon–stimulating acupressure massage point that you learned on page 175.

If you have a problem with chronic constipation, I recommend that you work with a qualified colon hygienist. Colonic irrigations not only clean out the waste, but they also exercise and tone the muscles of the colon, encouraging proper function. If you cannot find a colon therapist in your area, be sure to follow the dietary recommendations I have given, use intestinal cleansers, and give yourself at–home enemas when necessary to cleanse your colon.

Use the breathing exercises you have learned to breathe deeply into your abdomen. Notice any areas where you are tight and tense, and use your breath to open up and relax these areas. Yoga postures also help to release tension, as well as stimulating proper function of the abdominal organs.

Above all, learn to manage your stress. It is amazing how many people come into my office seeking help, and begin by denying that stress is contributing to their constipation problem. In my experience, constipation is usually caused by nutritional problems or emotional factors, or both. Once I have worked with clients on correcting their diet, if there is still a constipation problem, we begin to look at the impact of stress. Most people do not realize how much stress they have, and where they are storing it in their bodies. When we are under stress, many of us tend to tighten up in the abdominal area and lose touch with the proper functioning of the abdominal organs. Massage and deep breathing can help to increase your awareness of your body's stress patterns.

Sandy was a young mother who came to my office expressing great frustration with her constipation problem. Sandy was one of those people who denied stress. As we worked together on improving her diet, she came to trust me more and began to open up and talk about how stressful it was to be a mother. Her entire life was devoted to meeting the demands of her kids—

taking them one place after another, preparing meals for their differing fussy tastes, and maintaining a semblance of order at mealtimes. Somehow Sandy never found the time to take care of her own needs. We did a lot of work on her diet and colon cleansing, and Sandy was showing some improvement, but constipation was still a problem. We were really stumped, because we had tried just about everything. Then Sandy went away for a one–week vacation with her husband, leaving the kids at home in the care of a relative. Enjoying her holiday, Sandy ate everything she wanted, and to her amazement her bowel movements were regular. When she came back and told me what had happened, I realized that now we knew the real source of her problem. We discussed the possibilities, and came up with the idea that she and her husband should eat their evening meal alone, after the kids had been taken care of. No longer having to deal with the children at dinner, Sandy was able to relax while she ate. I was very gratified to see that this simple solution turned Sandy's problem around and ended her constipation. As with so many of my clients, the improvement in Sandy's bowel function was accompanied by an improvement in her sexual satisfaction. She had been so tight and uncomfortable in that part of her body that sex had never been pleasurable for her. Now, as she learned to let go of the stress in her abdominal organs, she also learned to relax and enjoy her sex life.

CONSTIPATION DO'S AND DON'TS

These tips can help you conquer constipation forever. Incorporate the Do's into your life, and you will begin to notice improved elimination patterns.

DO:

Eat your main meal early in the day—at mid-day, rather than in the evening.

Drink at least eight glasses of fluids each day.

Chew your food twenty to thirty times per mouthful.

Follow food-combining rules.

Use digestive enzymes when you miscombine foods or eat too much protein.

Use a fiber-rich intestinal cleanser.

Promote the friendly bacteria in your intestines by drinking Rejuvelac and using a Lactobacillus supplement.

Exercise regularly—walk, swim, use a trampoline, etc.

Use breathing exercises at least three times a week to relax the abdominal organs.

Practice yoga postures at least three times a week to tone and stimulate the digestive organs.

Practice slant-board exercises at least three times a week to rejuvenate the abdominal organs and strengthen the supporting muscles.

Take hot and cold sitz baths to stimulate the abdominal organs.

Use Hot Castor-Oil Abdominal Wraps to loosen up waste in the colon and relax the abdominal organs.

Use Tummy Massage to help elimination and locate tense areas.

Heed nature's call.

Establish the habit of moving your bowels at a specific time each day.

Use a footstool at the foot of your toilet to elevate your feet when moving your bowels.

Consult a sympathetic physician and a qualified colon hygienist; use colonic irrigations and enemas as needed to cleanse and tone the colon.

Take pride in proper bowel function.

Devote time each day to relaxing quietly and paying attention to managing your stress.

Get enough sleep—six to eight hours a day is the usual requirement for most people.

Think positive thoughts; use affirmations.

DON'T

Eat when you are upset.

Overeat.

Ignore food-combining principles.

Drink liquids with meals.

Use pharmaceutical laxatives.

Give in to worry or stress.

Suppress your feelings.

Put off going to the bathroom.

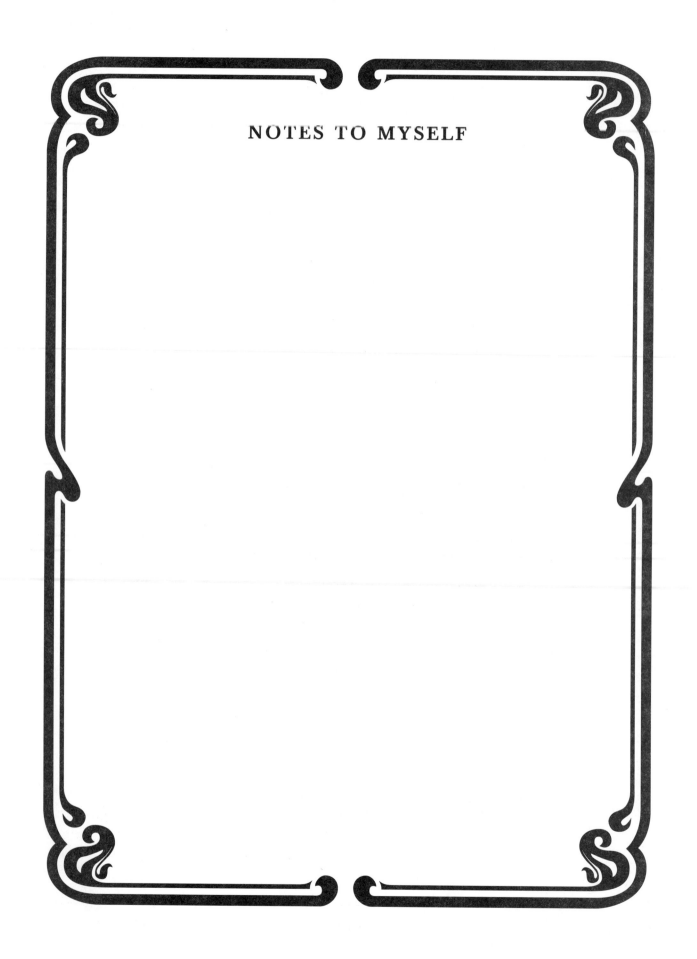

NOTES TO MYSELF

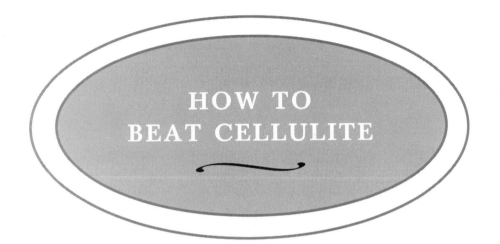

HOW TO
BEAT CELLULITE

*I*f you have been following the Cleansing and Rejuvenation Program, I am sure that you are feeling great about the weight you have lost. This is an ideal time to begin to attack your cellulite problem, if you have one, and to learn how to prevent the formation of cellulite in the future.

Cellulite (pronounced "sell–you–leet") is a term coined in the European health spas to describe the unsightly fatty deposits that do not go away even after extensive dieting and exercise. Cellulite tends to form in specific parts of the body–buttocks, upper thighs, knees, upper arms, and more rarely on the lower legs, abdomen, back of the neck, and ankles. Cellulite is easy to recognize once it has become fairly advanced. It has a characteristic doughy consistency and a lumpy, dimpled appearance, like cottage cheese. If you have it, you know exactly what I am talking about.

Cellulite is a very controversial subject in the United States. Although cellulite is still not recognized by the American medical establishment as a health problem, European doctors and health clinics have been treating it for years as a disease of the connective tissue, or "fat gone wrong." Most of my recommendations are based on the breakthrough research and treatment that has been done in Europe.

Cellulite is a gel–like substance made up of a combination of fat, waste material, and water that is trapped between strands of fibrous tissue just beneath the surface of the skin. Women tend to get cellulite much more frequently than men–about 80 percent of women have this problem to some degree. There are several reasons why cellulite is largely a feminine problem. To begin with, women have more fatty tissue than men. Cellulite forms in the layer of subcutaneous fatty tissue just below the skin; it is this tissue that provides the typical rounded feminine contours.

The female hormone estrogen also seems to contribute to the formation of cellulite. Women's bodies are flooded with estrogen before the menstrual period and sometimes also at ovulation. Just as estrogen is responsible for the psychological discomfort of premenstrual stress, it also encourages cellulite formation by promoting excess water retention in the tissues, leading to congestion of the lymphatic system in the legs and the groin region. Because the lymph system is responsible for removing protein waste from the body, this congestion causes the waste to be deposited in the surrounding connective tissue. The protein waste combines with fat cells, and the protein attracts water, forcing the cells to swell. The swelling causes the surrounding blood and lymph vessels to constrict, cutting down on circulation, and eventually the entire connective–tissue network enclosing the fat cells begins to atrophy and harden, forming a gelatin–like network with pockets of fat cells puffed up with water.

Out of desperation, trying to rid their bodies of these unsightly bulges, women go on crash diets. Their bodies produce enzymes to break down body fat for energy, but these enzymes cannot reach the stagnant cellulite deposits of fat, water, and waste, because the circulation to these areas is already impaired. As a result, the fat melts away from other parts of the body, such as the breasts and the facial tissues, creating the haggard, aged appearance that is so characteristic of crash dieters.

The formation of cellulite is very closely connected to constipation and the resultant toxicity. The more toxic waste that is allowed to accumulate in the body, the greater is the chance that it will find its way into the subcutaneous fatty tissue and get trapped in stagnant cellulite deposits. This is an excellent reason to avoid all foods containing chemicals and pesticides and hard–to–digest refined and processed food, and to observe the rules of food combining, so that wastes are flushed out of the system as rapidly as possible.

The renowned French herbalist and healer Maurice Messegue did extensive experiments on cellulite control with women from all over Europe. He found that it was only when these women gave up eating foods that contained pesticides and other chemicals that they were able to begin to reduce the cellulite in their bodies. Such chemicals create extra stress on the liver, preventing it from doing its job of breaking up fatty deposits and removing excess estrogen and other hormones from the body. Excess estrogen increases the tendency to water retention, promoting the formation of new cellulite.

GLA and EPA not only keep your skin, hair, and nails strong and healthy, but they also help to prevent the formation of harmful fatty deposits in the blood vessels and to burn the subcutaneous fat that can provide a home for waste material and turn into cellulite.

Our sedentary lifestyle also contributes to the formation of cellulite. Prolonged sitting causes the blockage of blood and lymph circulation in the thighs and buttocks. If you have a sedentary job, it is particularly important to get regular exercise to promote circulation in these cellulite–prone areas. Do slant–board activities to promote drainage of lymph and blood, use

CELLULITE CONTROL DIET

Proper digestion and elimination of toxins are the keys to banishing cellulite from your body. Make a commitment to eat the clean and clear Foods to Eat and beware of the Foods to Avoid, and you can take control of your figure problems.

FOODS TO EAT:

Organically grown fresh fruits and vegetables—no chemicals or pesticides
Whole grains
Fresh juices
Fibrous foods in general
Sea vegetables and other iodine–rich foods
At least eight glasses of fluids each day–juices, herb teas, Hydrating Drink, purified water, broth
GLA oil in salad dressing and GLA-EPA supplement
Supplements: aloe vera juice, liquid minerals, digestive enzymes, vitamin B6 for detoxifying excess estrogen, intestinal cleanser
Liver Flush drinks for special periodic cleansing

FOODS TO AVOID:

Processed foods—synthetics, preservatives. additives
Nonorganic meats or poultry
Fish from shallow or possibly polluted waters
Fatty foods
Tap water
Sugar
Salt
Bread
White flour
Salted snack foods
Fried foods
Candies, cookies, and pastries
Cheese
Excessive animal protein
Excessive alcohol
Excessive caffeine

full–body massage and lymph massage to aid the flushing of wastes, and practice yoga postures that stimulate circulation and tone the muscles that control elimination. Detoxifying Baths such as those on pages 152 through 158, Herbal Steams, Hot Castor–Oil Abdominal Wraps on page 186, Sitz Baths on page 155, and Foot Baths on page 161 also help to promote circulation and drain waste from the lymphatic system. Daily skin brushing described on page 144 is an essential routine for cellulite control, removing waste from the skin so that it is fresh each day to do its job of eliminating the body's debris.

In addition to the general measures that you are learning in the Cleansing and Rejuvenation Program, I am now going to give you specific techniques for dealing with any cellulite in your body. Many massage therapists use a specialized form of massage to help break up fatty cellulite deposits and bring circulation into the affected areas to carry away the waste that has been trapped there. You can do the same kind of massage yourself on a regular basis to help rid your body of these unsightly deposits.

Before I show you how to do a cellulite self–massage, you need to know where cellulite is located in your body, and what kind of cellulite it is. The Cellulite Self–Exam will enable you to take stock of your cellulite situation. Do not despair if you find deposits of cellulite. My 21–Day Program is designed to help you break up this cellulite and flush the debris out of your body, as well as discourage the formation of new cellulite.

CELLULITE SELF–EXAM

To locate cellulite deposits on your body, stand undressed before a full length mirror. If you do not see any obvious areas of ripples, lumps, or cottage–cheese skin, try squeezing the tissues of your upper thigh between the thumb and index finger, or between the palms of both hands. If cellulite is present, the skin will dimple and have a characteristic quilted appearance. Try this squeezing test on all the areas of your body where cellulite is most likely to occur–the outer parts of the upper thighs, the buttocks, the inner knees, the upper arms, the abdomen–unless you can actually see the dimpling effect without squeezing. Not every fatty area will dimple, only those areas with toxic cellulite.

There are two kinds of cellulite, solid and soft. Solid or firm cellulite generally appears on women who are in good physical condition. You may notice that even female marathon runners with muscular, sinewy legs may show the telltale signs of puckered skin on their outer thighs. People with solid cellulite generally do not have much fatty tissue, and cannot easily lift the cellulite away from the underlying muscle. Squeezing or pinching the skin in solid cellulite areas may produce pain or sensitivity. The skin in these areas is generally dry and sometimes rough, due to poor nourishment, and it may have stretch marks.

Soft cellulite is not as concentrated or compact as solid cellulite. It tends to occupy large areas, and to hang loosely, shaking with every body movement. Soft cellulite tends to affect women with poor muscle tone and soft skin; they may have been active in the past but have become inactive for some time. People who go on crash diets often end up with soft cellulite because the yo–yo weight changes cause the tissues to lose their elasticity.

After looking at yourself in the mirror and trying the squeeze test, you probably have a good idea of whether you have any cellulite, and whether it is solid or soft. To tell how advanced a case of cellulite you have, notice whether there is any sensitivity on touching or pinching the skin in the cellulite areas. The more advanced the cellulite, the more tender and painful it is when pinched or squeezed.

CELLULITE MASSAGE OIL

If you have cellulite, prepare this aromatic oil to use for the Cellulite Massage below. Massage the oil liberally into any areas affected by cellulite to help break up the fatty deposits and mobilize the waste.

1 ounce olive oil
1 ounce almond oil
1 ounce peanut oil
12 drops rosemary essential oil
12 drops geranium oil

Combine all ingredients and store in an airtight container.

In addition to the moisturizing and beautifying benefits of the vegetable oils, the essential oils in this recipe have special detoxifying properties. Rosemary oil stimulates the function of the liver as it breaks down fat, regulates hormone balance, and synthesizes new proteins to build healthy skin. Geranium oil helps to maintain proper hormone balance, and is used to relieve

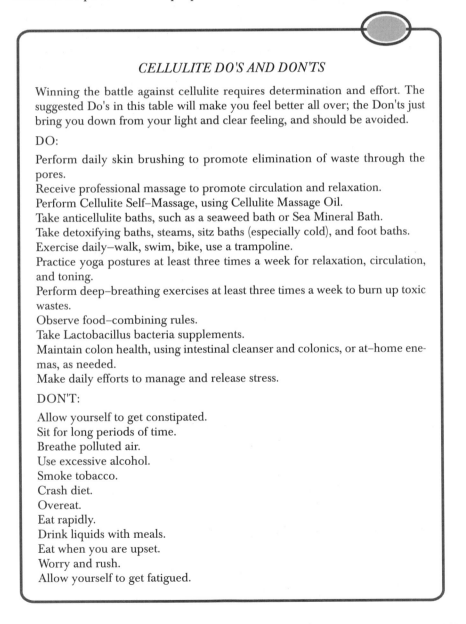

CELLULITE DO'S AND DON'TS

Winning the battle against cellulite requires determination and effort. The suggested Do's in this table will make you feel better all over; the Don'ts just bring you down from your light and clear feeling, and should be avoided.

DO:

Perform daily skin brushing to promote elimination of waste through the pores.
Receive professional massage to promote circulation and relaxation.
Perform Cellulite Self–Massage, using Cellulite Massage Oil.
Take anticellulite baths, such as a seaweed bath or Sea Mineral Bath.
Take detoxifying baths, steams, sitz baths (especially cold), and foot baths.
Exercise daily—walk, swim, bike, use a trampoline.
Practice yoga postures at least three times a week for relaxation, circulation, and toning.
Perform deep–breathing exercises at least three times a week to burn up toxic wastes.
Observe food–combining rules.
Take Lactobacillus bacteria supplements.
Maintain colon health, using intestinal cleanser and colonics, or at–home enemas, as needed.
Make daily efforts to manage and release stress.

DON'T:

Allow yourself to get constipated.
Sit for long periods of time.
Breathe polluted air.
Use excessive alcohol.
Smoke tobacco.
Crash diet.
Overeat.
Eat rapidly.
Drink liquids with meals.
Eat when you are upset.
Worry and rush.
Allow yourself to get fatigued.

the excessive fluid retention that produces premenstrual stress. They stimulate the lymphatic system and aid the elimination of waste and fluids.

CELLULITE MASSAGE

Please understand that cellulite massage by itself will not miraculously make your cellulite problem disappear. To get rid of cellulite, you must make a serious commitment to the Clean and Clear Diet, and to the entire program I am recommending. Only if you have laid the groundwork by doing everything else right will the cellulite massage be able to help, and you must do the self–massage diligently and regularly to break up the cellulite deposits.

Your cellulite massage will be concentrated on the areas where you have identified cellulite. You can do it any time you want–during your bath, or whenever you have a few minutes–to help increase the blood and lymph flow to these circulation–starved areas, break down the cellulite, and move the resultant waste out of your body.

Do not press too hard when doing a cellulite massage. Begin with moderate pressure and increase only as you know you can tolerate it without bruising or discomfort.

Before you do your first cellulite massage, make up a batch of Cellulite Massage Oil, above. This special, fragrant formulation not only lubricates the skin but also penetrates the tissue, helping to promote the removal of toxins. Warm some of the Cellulite Massage Oil in your hands. Then begin by stroking lightly over the cellulite areas, to prepare the skin for the movements that follow. Continue to apply Cellulite Massage Oil throughout this massage whenever necessary to lubricate and penetrate the skin. Using the flat of your hand with the fingers curved around the body part, use long, light, smooth, sliding strokes, always moving toward the heart. Stroke upward on your legs, over the hips and buttocks, and in the same clockwise direction over the tummy that you used in the Tummy Massage on page 187, working from the navel to the right side, then up and over the navel to the left, down and below the navel and up again on the right side. If you have cellulite on your upper arms or upper torso, stroke upward into the armpit and down the chest toward the heart.

The next movements you use depend on what type of cellulite you have. If you have soft cellulite that you can grasp between your fingers or between your palms, grab a hunk of cellulite tissue, lift it away from the underlying muscles, and squeeze it firmly. You can do this with your fingers or with the whole hand, depending on how large an area you are working on. Using your fingers or whole hand, lift the cellulite tissue and squeeze, lift and squeeze, working all over the area where you see the cellulite. In areas like the inner knee or the upper arm, squeezing with the fingers is most effective. Lift and squeeze with the whole hand to work on the larger cellulite areas over the hips and buttocks. Work upward from the upper thighs and over the hips. When you massage the leg below the upper thigh, rest your foot on a stool or the edge of the tub, or sit with your knee bent, to relax the muscles.

If you can lift large areas of cellulite tissue with both hands, wring it between your hands and twist it around. Squeeze it to break up the deposits inside and encourage circulation. If you cannot pick up the flesh, just squeeze and wring the tissues between both hands. This is no time to be gentle! Squeeze that cellulite out of your body.

If you have solid cellulite, you may not be able to lift the tissue away from the underlying structure at all, and you will need to employ crushing movements to break up the cellulite deposits and encourage circulation. For solid cellulite, do the crushing movements directly after the initial light stroking. Bunch your hands into fists and, with the knuckles, crush the cellulite areas with a circular motion. Go ahead, take out all your aggressions on those bulges! These crushing movements are very effective for the hips, upper thighs, and tummy.

End your massage with deep, firm stroking. Use full pressure, going in the direction of the heart. Use the flat of your hand, with the fingers and thumb curved around the part of the body you are massaging, and slide your hands in long, deep strokes, exerting pressure. Stroke toward the heart—up the legs and hips, and clockwise over the tummy. Firm stroking promotes the circulation of blood and lymph and helps to drain away the waste matter that has been released by the massage movements.

You may have noticed that my recommendations of a Cellulite Control Diet, as well as the Cellulite Do's and Don'ts, are very similar to those for controlling constipation on page 194, except that the cellulite control recommendations focus specifically on eliminating toxic substances and balancing hormone function. This similarity is not coincidental. Proper elimination helps prevent the buildup of fatty deposits and removes the toxic wastes that ultimately get trapped in fatty tissue to create cellulite.

By making a strong commitment to observe these recommendations, you will begin to win your battle against cellulite. It can be a long process. Use affirmations to maintain a positive attitude and help control stress, since anxiety, worry and feeling bad about yourself can cause your muscles to tighten and impair circulation in the very areas where you want to flush the waste away. Each time you do a Cellulite Self–Massage, remind yourself that your efforts are going to pay off with smooth new contours and healthy, glowing, youthful skin.

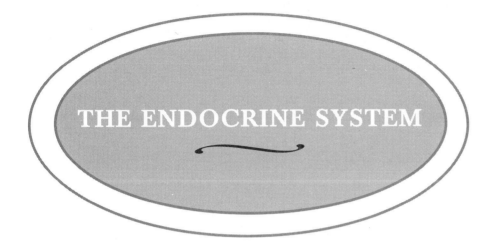

THE ENDOCRINE SYSTEM

A Support To Your Vitality

Scientists tell us that we are as young as our glands. Your body's endocrine glands secrete hormones directly into the bloodstream and lymph system, exerting wide-ranging effects on other glands and on virtually every organ in the body. Many of the rejuvenating benefits of my 21-Day Program come from providing your endocrine glands with what they need to function properly—not just specific foods and nutrients, but also freedom from stress, adequate exercise, and cleansing of the systems of elimination.

Researchers are learning more about the endocrine glands all the time, and some are understood better than others. The pituitary gland, located deep in the brain, regulates the functioning of the glandular system of the entire body. The pineal gland, also located in the brain, is still little understood. It has been associated in esoteric literature with the "third eye," and appears to be sensitive to light. The thyroid, located in the neck, is the gland most directly involved in regulating metabolism, which affects your weight. It is responsible for the burning of fat and it also controls the activity of the sex glands. The parathyroids, attached to the thyroid, regulate calcium metabolism and control the activity of lymph in neutralizing certain toxins. The thymus, located in the chest, is also little understood, but it is known to be responsible for producing crucial disease-fighting white cells in the

ROYAL JELLY: THE YOUTH FOOD

Royal jelly is the miraculous substance that is fed to the chosen female bee, transforming her into the queen of the hive and making her extremely fertile. Royal jelly extends the bee's normal life span of a few weeks to more than five years. Rich in B vitamins, amino acids, and minerals, royal jelly is a popular rejuvenation and nutritional aid in China and Japan. You can purchase it either in capsule form or in a honey base and add it to your drinks as a sweetener.

immune system. The pancreas not only produces digestive enzymes, but specialized parts of the pancreas also function as an endocrine gland, producing the insulin that regulates your body's use of sugar. The adrenal glands, sitting on top of the kidneys, produce two kinds of substances. The inner part of the adrenals produces adrenaline, the hormone that prepares the body for vigorous activity in response to stress. The outer part of the adrenal glands produces the adrenocorticoids, powerful hormones that, when present in excess, are largely responsible for the organ damage that comes from prolonged stress. The sex glands include the prostate in men and the ovaries in women. When levels of sex hormones diminish, many signs of aging tend to set in.

REJUVENATION THROUGH GLANDULAR HEALTH

Some of your glands require specific foods or nutrients to stay healthy. The thyroid gland requires iodine to maintain balanced activity. Sea vegetables are particularly rich in iodine. Many recipes are provided using sea vegetables on pages 106 through 107, such as the Hijiki Stir–Fry, which are an excellent food for stimulating proper thyroid function and helping to regulate your metabolism, your weight, and your sex glands.

Many vitamins are important for maintaining glandular health. Vitamin C helps all your glands to work at the peak of their capacity, as well as protecting your body against aging in general. Vitamin C is known to be necessary for adequate sex–hormone production, and to help the adrenal glands produce their hormones. The bioflavonoids, including rutin, work to increase the biological effect of vitamin C and help to overcome premature aging. Vitamin A is another all–purpose rejuvenating and protective vitamin. Vitamin A deficiency has been specifically shown to impair the ability of the thymus gland to produce the crucial disease–fighting T lymphocytes of the immune system. It also aids communication between your cells, protecting against the growth of mutated cells.

The B–complex vitamins are extremely important for glandular health. Vitamin B1, or thiamine, is known as an age–fighting vitamin, and it helps the pituitary gland to regulate the sex organs. Pantothenic acid protects against stress, and has been known to help women delay the onset of menopause. PABA and folic acid, two other B vitamins, are reported to help keep the sex glands functioning effectively. Vitamin B6, or pyridoxine, helps protect against impotence in men, and against PMS in women, and specifically helps the liver to convert potentially harmful excess estrogen into harmless substances. In fact, all the B vitamins help to support the detoxifying function of the liver and help the body overcome the effects of stress. Obviously, it is a good idea to take a high-potency vitamin–B complex supplement to promote glandular rejuvenation.

Lecithin is a very important food for glandular rejuvenation. It is present in all the endocrine glands, especially in the pituitary, the pineal, and the male and female sex glands, and it is an important component of semen. Lecithin is claimed to help improve virility and to prevent impotence. After you have finished doing the 21–Day Program, please continue to sprinkle granulated lecithin on your salads or soups and add it to your protein drinks to ensure an adequate supply of this life extending nutrient.

Vitamin E protects against the aging effects of damaging free radicals in the body. In animal studies, vitamin E has been found to be essential to proper function of the reproductive glands.

As you see how important all these vitamins are to the health of your glands, you will understand why I recommend on page 72 that you take a comprehensive regimen of vitamin supplements every day.

Of the minerals, I particularly want to call attention to the importance of zinc. Many male sexual problems, including prostatitis and impotence, can often be traced to zinc deficiency. Seafood, especially shellfish, is an excellent source of zinc, but beware of possible contamination in shellfish. Nuts, legumes, and whole grains are other good zinc sources, and pumpkin seeds are very rich in zinc. A zinc supplement may prove helpful for men who are having sexual problems. Zinc also is healthful for the immune system.

One of the herbs most widely associated with rejuvenating the endocrine system is Wild Yam. This popular herb is known to contain the natural precursors of the adrenal hormones, and its long term use can be highly beneficial for anyone in very stressful conditions. These hormone precursors are natural building blocks which the body can utilize while the gland is being restored to its natural function. Wild Yam is also known for its ability to strengthen, tone, and stimulate the secretive functions of the liver. This important organ is intimately involved in all bodily functions and the health of all tissues. I have written more about the uses of Wild Yam for hormone balancing on page 216.

Far too many Americans develop diabetes in middle age, especially if they are overweight. Many people do not realize that this is partially due to an imbalance of the endocrine system. Diet is undoubtedly one of the causative factors. The incidence of diabetes tends to be measurably higher in populations eating a "civilized" modern diet low in fiber and high in refined sugar and starch than among native populations eating high–fiber diets based on whole, unrefined foods. Once diabetes develops, it not only limits what foods you can eat for the rest of your life–restricting you of necessity to a healthy Clean and Clear Diet–but it also dramatically increases the risk of heart disease. To avoid this terribly destructive disease, keep your weight within a normal range.

To keep your glands young, it is very important that you maintain a positive mental attitude. The health of your adrenal glands, and hence of your entire body, depends on your ability to control stress. When you are under stress, the adrenals first secrete adrenaline, and then, as the stress reaction continues, they begin to secrete cortisol, a compound that can have a damaging effect on all the organs of the body. Certain kinds of stimulants such as caffeine can produce chronic stress on the adrenal glands. This is one of the very good reasons to keep your overall caffeine consumption to a minimum.

If you would like professional guidance in evaluating your glandular health and establishing a program for glandular rejuvenation, I recommend that you contact a holistic doctor. Please consult the Referral Guide on page 230 for assistance in locating a qualified doctor in your area. These doctors are skilled at evaluating your glandular functioning and prescribing special high–dose vitamin–supplement programs to correct any possible imbalances.

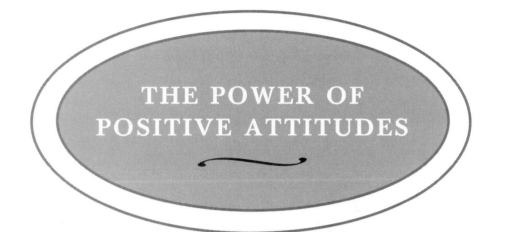

THE POWER OF
POSITIVE ATTITUDES

*A*s you begin to experience the clear, light, clean feeling that comes
with a thorough cleansing of your systems of elimination, you will
also begin to realize that a polluted body can affect the way you think and
feel. Truly, a polluted body produces a polluted mind.

If you have already done the cleansing phase of the 21–Day Program, I
am certain that it has left you feeling better than you have felt for a very long
time. If you have had any symptoms from cleansing reactions–troubled skin,
aches and pains, mild headache, and so forth–remember that they are just
part of getting better. In fact, the stronger your cleansing reactions are, the
more toxins you had to eliminate from your body, and the healthier you will
be as a result. All the suggestions I have given you in this program about
drinking lots of fluids, getting plenty of exercise, rest and relaxation, should
have helped to minimize any cleansing symptoms. Remember to look at
these symptoms from a positive, releasing point of view, and don't sabotage
your hard work by becoming discouraged, or by using chemical remedies
that will introduce toxins into your system, bringing you down from your
high, positive feeling.

Just as a congested, toxic body will produce cloudy, negative thoughts, it
is equally true that negative thoughts and attitudes can adversely affect your
body. Folk wisdom has always taught that negative thinking and stress can
lead to illness. Now, medical research is beginning to show exactly how this
happens. The new field of psychoneuroimmunology studies the interactions
between thinking (psycho), the brain and central nervous system (neuro),
and the immune system (immunology). We now understand that stress caus-

es the body to produce potent hormones that damage the organs and can lead to disease. Stress can also suppress the proper functioning of the immune system.

In the 1960's, medical researchers Thomas Holmes and Richard Rahe devised a scale for evaluating significant life changes, both pleasant and unpleasant, that produce stress. Different life changes were given different scores, with the highest score being assigned to the death of a spouse. Examples of other stress–causing events include being fired from a job, retirement, a change in residence, travel, and marriage. Generally, the higher a person's Life Change Score for a specific period of time, the greater would be the likelihood that he or she developed a serious illness following these life changes.

We now know that the relationship between stressful events and illness is not quite that simple. It turns out that some people, rather than being made sick by stress, are actually spurred on to higher levels of performance. Why are some people made ill by stress, while others thrive on it? In an attempt to answer this question, psychologist Suzanne Kobasa studied executives at the Illinois Bell Telephone Company during the stressful period of the AT&T divestiture. She found that the stress–resistant executives had certain characteristics in common, which she labeled challenge, commitment, and control. Challenge means that the executives who remained healthy were able to view the potentially threatening situation as a challenge–a stimulus to creativity and high performance. Commitment means that those who successfully survived stress felt deeply committed to their work, their families, their personal well–being, and other important values. Finally, the control factor meant that the healthy executives saw themselves as being in charge of their lives, instead of feeling they were victims of outside circumstances.

The point of this research is that it is not stress itself that can make you ill, but your attitude toward it. This means that by learning to relax and be flexible in the face of change, you can protect yourself to a very large extent from the ill effects of stress. This is exactly what I have been talking about when I say that your attitude affects the way you feel and look. By programming your mind with positive messages, you will be able to cope with stress, your body will work much better, and you will greatly reduce the danger of developing a serious illness in the future.

Think for a moment about any feelings that have come up while you have been on this program, and about how you can use the attitudes described as challenge, commitment, and control to keep you on track. Think also about the things that are causing stress in your life right now, and about how affirmations embodying challenge, commitment, and control can help you to cope better. The more you program yourself with a positive diet for the mind, the more you will be able to sail successfully through the potentially distressing events in your daily life.

Take out your journal now, and write some affirmations that seem appropriate for you. Think in terms of the qualities of challenge, commitment, and control. Possible affirmations might be: "I am committed to making myself as healthy as I can be, so that I can be better for the people I love"; "I have the power to control my diet by choosing the foods that are best for me"; or "I welcome the challenge of walking or bicycling instead of using my car." Use affirmations embodying challenge, commitment, and control every day. You will be surprised at how much more powerful this diet for the mind will make you feel.

USING AFFIRMATIONS: A CLEANSING DIET FOR THE MIND

Perhaps The Cleansing and Rejuvenation Program is a completely new experience for you. You may find it difficult to let go of foods that have always been sources of comfort and security. An excellent tool to help you hold your resolve is to use affirmations every day. Affirmations are simply positive statements that keep you focused on your purpose and help to remind you that you are doing something wonderful for your body. You first used affirmations on this program when you repeated positive phrases such as "Peace, harmony, and well–being," on your daily walks. Now, I will show you some other ways to use these powerful self–programming tools.

Every time you sit down to eat a meal, use an affirmation to dedicate the food to your well–being. In your mind or out loud, say something like, "I am giving my body a wonderful gift by following this program," or "I am rejuvenating my body with this wonderful cleansing food." When you wake up in the morning, use affirmations to create a positive, optimistic frame of mind. Tell yourself something like, "My body feels alive and wonderful. I feel healthy and rejuvenated." When you are tempted to stray from your diet or to ignore other elements of this program, use an affirmation to keep yourself on track, such as, "I release all negative thoughts," or "I will feel wonderful after I do my exercise."

As you cleanse your body, negative thoughts and emotions may come up. Use affirmations to reprogram your unconscious mind, to truly express love for yourself and recognize that you are taking care of yourself. When you experience negative thoughts or disturbing emotions, use an affirmation such as, "I welcome the opportunity to cleanse myself of old negative feelings."

Fill your journal with affirmations and bring it with you to work, so that you can reinforce your resolve during the day. Filling your mind with positive thoughts actually changes the way you feel. Try it–affirmations are a powerful tool and a wonderful habit to develop. I have found that even if initially I don't really feel it as truth, as I continue to repeat the thought, I will slowly change my innate thinking. It works if you allow it to!

*BOOKS ON
POSITIVE THINKING*

Read more about the power of positive thinking! Some of my favorite books include :

Ageless Body, Timeless Mind *by Deepak Chopra, M.D. (Harmony Books)*

Perfect Health *by Deepak Chopra, M.D. (Random House)*

You Can Heal Your Life *by Louise Hay (Coleman)*

Heal Your Body *by Louise Hay (Hay House)*

NOTES TO MYSELF

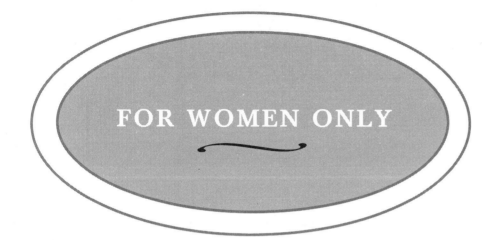

FOR WOMEN ONLY

*I*n native cultures, even today, the menstrual period is considered a powerful rite of passage and a cleansing process. In fact, the cyclical cleansing through the loss of menstrual blood may be one reason that women live longer than men. I particularly like the Native American traditions of honoring the "moon time." Among many American Indian tribes, women retire each month to "moon lodges." This does not mean that they are stuck away somewhere, as people often believe. Rather, the women are given the gift of a quiet, peaceful several days when they are not expected to carry out their usual chores. In the moon lodge, the women relax and meditate, often coming away with visions that help to guide the future activities of the tribe.

Native Americans understand that the menstrual cycle is linked with the phases of the moon. The full moon is the time of ovulation, when energy is more externally directed, and the new moon is the time of menstruation, a time when energy draws within. Many women, even in modern society, find that personal and spiritual issues that do not come to the surface during the rest of the month seem to become more pronounced around the menstrual time. As you become more aware of how your cycles affect your mind and body, you can use this special time of the month to gain insights about important personal issues.

Several years ago, my sister and a friend developed an idea for a retreat center especially for women during their "moon time," where they would be able to get away for a few days and be taken care of. When I told my sister recently about the Indian moon lodges, she was delighted to realize that her idea had really arisen from a need that all women feel for a different pace during the menstrual period. It is important for women to recognize that demanding, high pressure schedules should not be maintained throughout the entire month. While you may not be able to afford the luxury of getting away on a monthly basis, you can create a protective haven for yourself during your own cycles. During my menstrual period, I schedule fewer clients, knowing that my lighter work load will give me more quiet time to myself.

The first step in turning your menstrual period into a beneficial, cleansing time is to come to know your cycles. It amazes me how many women I work with are not aware of their "moon cycles," and of the changes that take place in their bodies, their dietary needs, and their moods. When they begin to keep track, most women find that they have their period around either the full or the new moon, although the cycle may change over time. By learning to recognize your cycle, you have another opportunity to gain insight about your body. If you are not already doing so, begin to log your menstrual cycle on your personal calendar. Note in your calendar also any symptoms that are associated with the premenstrual period, or with the onset of menstruation. Do you become bloated or constipated before your period? Do you notice premenstrual tension and stress? Do you sleep less or more than usual? As you become more aware of the rhythms of your body, you will know when to use natural interventions to make this a more pleasant time for yourself, and you will be able to deal more appropriately with your feelings, your work schedule, and your relationships.

It is also important to know when you ovulate. Regardless of the length of your entire menstrual cycle, ovulation normally occurs about fourteen days before your next menstrual period begins. We have other ways also of identifying when ovulation occurs. The basal body temperature, or the lowest daily temperature that the body reaches during waking hours, drops just before ovulation, and then at ovulation rises steadily for the next three days or so, remaining elevated until menstruation begins. Women practicing natural birth control use this basal-temperature method to help predict the fertile days of their monthly cycle. Another method used in natural birth control is to observe the changes in the cervical mucus and vaginal discharges throughout the month. The normal vaginal discharge between menstruation and ovulation is white, cloudy, or yellowish, and thick and sticky. A few days before ovulation, the discharge increases in volume and becomes clear and slippery like raw egg white. Classes in natural birth control and fertility awareness, available through women's clinics and Planned Parenthood, can help you to become more aware of your ovulation and menstrual cycle, so that your monthly mood and body changes will no longer take you by surprise.

In our society, PMS, or premenstrual syndrome, has come to be viewed as a disorder that encompasses a wide range of symptoms such as mood swings, headache, bloating, breast tenderness, irritability, and depression. It is not so well known that some researchers have found that women also exhibit positive changes during this premenstrual time, such as greater ability to concentrate, and increased creativity and assertiveness. Such changes are due to the interplay of hormones. Before the menstrual period, excess estrogen overbalances progesterone, producing the typical PMS symptoms. The body is then flooded with progesterone when menstruation begins, and the symptoms are alleviated.

I find that if I follow the Clean and Clear Diet as described on pages 61 through 77 and practice food rotation as explained on pages 75 through 76, my premenstrual symptoms are diminished almost entirely. Most of my female clients find the same. The liver is responsible for removing excess estrogen from the system. By reducing the burden on your liver produced by improper diet, you enable it to regulate your delicate hormonal balance and detoxify the excess estrogen. A special program of supplements can also help you to prepare for your menstrual period and reduce the symptoms of PMS. Interestingly, the same healthy program will also prepare you for a healthier, more symptom free, menopause.

Smooth-Cycle Checklist

In addition to practicing proper food combining and taking your usual supplements, begin to make these special alterations in your diet and supplement program about three to seven days before your menstrual period is due, and continue until the end of menstruation. If you still experience uncomfortable premenstrual or menstrual symptoms, try beginning earlier the next month, until you find the right time to provide your body with this extra nutritional support.

Supplements

* Take 50 to 150 milligrams of vitamin B6, along with a complete B complex, to help control premenstrual mood swings and other emotional problems, and support the liver in detoxifying excess estrogen.

* Take a special PMS formula, available in health-food stores. Such a formula may contain enough vitamin B6 or other nutrients that you do not need to take these as separate supplements.

* Take a multi-phase digestive enzyme to help prevent constipation and reduce the toxic burden on your liver. (Digestive Enzymes are described on page 74).

* Take a Wild Yam supplement to balance your hormones. (I describe this herbal remedy on page 216).

* If your PMS symptoms are not alleviated by supplements alone, consult your doctor about applying progesterone cream to your skin. (It is available as both a cream and roll–on). It is also very effective in alleviating cramping when applied directly to the abdomen at the time that the symptom appears.

Diet

* Cut down on red meat, because its high fat content increases stress on the liver.

* Eliminate caffeine, because it depletes B vitamins needed to help the liver break down estrogen.

WILD YAM: A "FOUNTAIN OF YOUTH"

Wild Yam is valued both in the herbal and scientific communities for its powerful effect on regulating hormone production. Though primarily regarded as a progesterone producing herb, it acts to regulate the ratio of progesterone to estrogen in the system. According to Dr. John Lee M.D., an authority on natural hormonal therapies, the progesterone taken from the Wild Yam is nearly identical to what the body produces; the body easily converts it into the identical molecule. It is most helpful in balancing symptoms from PMS, perimenopause and menopause.

Wild Yam is also known to contain the natural precursors of the adrenal hormones, including natural cortisones. The long term use of this herb can be highly beneficial for anyone in very stressful conditions. These hormone precursors are natural building blocks which the body can utilize while the gland is being restored to its natural function.

Wild Yam is also known for its ability to strengthen, tone, and stimulate the secretive functions of the liver. This most important organ is intimately involved in all bodily functions and the health of all tissues.

It is now finally available in a form that can survive the digestive process and deliver it as needed to the endocrine system.

* Eliminate sugar and alcohol, because they aggravate blood–sugar reactions and depression.

* Be sure to drink at least eight glasses of water daily, to keep the system hydrated and flush away toxins that may produce symptoms.

* To prevent bloating and constipation before your period, drink one cup of Diuretic Tea daily. Continue until your period begins.

* Reduce your salt intake to discourage water retention.

* Eat watermelon to help flush water out of your tissues.

* Eat extra cucumbers for their diuretic effect.

* Eat extra garlic to support liver function and protect against vaginal infections.

* Eat sea vegetables to help regulate your hormone balance.

* To control sweet cravings before your period, try eating additional protein. You may need to increase your protein intake as early as ovulation time.

* To relieve breast tenderness, try eliminating hard–to–digest foods such as bread and cheese.

Moon–Time Tonic Tea

Herbs are a wonderful aid in preventing uncomfortable premenstrual and menstrual symptoms such as emotional ups and downs, cramps, sore breasts and muscles. Prepare a batch of Moon–Time Tonic Tea blend as follows.

> 1/2 cup red raspberry leaf
> 1/4 cup licorice root, shredded or broken into
> pieces
> 1/4 cup squaw vine
> 1/2 cup chamomile

Combine all the herbs thoroughly and store in an airtight container. For each cup of tea, add one teaspoon of the herbal blend to one cup of boiling water. Cover and steep for thirty minutes. Strain the tea into a thermos or other container and drink it one cup at a time according to the schedule that follows.

Begin to drink this Moon–Time Tonic Tea about three to seven days before your next period–before you usually experience the onset of symptoms. Drink two cups of the tea each day, between meals, until your period begins. During your menstrual period, continue to drink it, then discontinue until before your next period. If you use this Moon–Time Tonic Tea as directed over a few months' time, you should begin to notice an easing of premenstrual symptoms. If the above schedule does not control your symptoms, begin drinking the tea earlier in the month.

The combination of herbs in this tonic are specifically targeted at the discomforts that may arise during the menstrual cycle. Chamomile is very soothing to the nervous system, and chaparral assists in the cleansing and detoxifying process. Squaw vine and red raspberry leaf are traditional "female remedies" that help to balance the female system, promote uterine activity, and reduce menstrual cramps. Licorice root assists hormonal balancing and imparts a lively, sweet flavor to the tea, helping to overcome a craving for sweets.

Moon–Time Movements and Massage

During your premenstrual and menstrual time, nurture yourself with yoga, breathing exercises, and massage. A yoga exercise that is particularly beneficial for the pelvic organs is the YOGA ARCH POSE VARIATIONS on page 124. Practice this exercise daily during your menstrual period to alleviate cramping and tone your female organs.

Self–massage is also helpful during this time. Beginning about three days before your period, do the TUMMY MASSAGE I describe on page 187 to help prevent constipation. To relieve premenstrual bloating, menstrual cramps, or achy legs, massage around your ankles and lower legs to increase circulation, relieve congestion, and soothe the female organs. The LOWER–BODY LYMPH MASSAGE on page 162, accompanied by a hot foot soak on page 162, is great for relieving lymphatic congestion and cramping.

The SOOTHING "HOT SEAT" BATH on page 155, with essential oils, is a great remedy for menstrual cramps. Take one as often as you wish during your menstrual period to help energize the pelvic organs and relieve pain. Add six drops of lavender, chamomile, or marjoram essential oil.

The HOT CASTOR-OIL ABDOMINAL WRAP on page 186 is a great remedy for many menstrual discomforts. It helps to alleviate constipation and promote cleansing, relieves cramping, and is a wonderful way to achieve deep relaxation when you feel irritability creeping up before or during your moon time.

Inner Beauty Douche

The risk of vaginal infections changes in relation to the menstrual cycle. The vagina becomes more alkaline at ovulation and menstruation, and that is when vaginitis and symptoms of yeast infections tend to appear. The vagina is a self-cleansing organ, so I do not recommend douching as a matter of routine. If, however, you have a tendency to develop these problems, use the Inner Beauty Douche at the end of the menstrual period to re-acidify the vagina.

> 1 quart REJUVELAC (page 88)
> 1 quart MOON-TIME TONIC TEA (page 217)
> 2 tablespoons apple-cider vinegar
> 2 tablespoons liquid acidophilus

Combine the above ingredients and warm them if necessary to a comfortable temperature for douching.

Sterilize your douche apparatus by filling it with warm water and adding about one teaspoon of alcohol. Run this mixture through the apparatus to kill any lingering germs. Then fill it with the douche mixture and douche very slowly and gently, so that you do not force bacteria up into the uterus.

You can use this Inner Beauty Douche at ovulation also, if you tend to get vaginal infections at that time. At ovulation time, omit the Moon-Time Tonic from the recipe and use two quarts of Rejuvelac with the apple-cider vinegar and liquid acidophilus.

If you do not have time to prepare the Rejuvelac and the Moon-Time Tonic Tea, you may simply use the apple cider vinegar and liquid acidophilus.

Moon-Time Cleansing Program

If you are troubled by discomfort during the premenstrual or menstrual period, the Moon-Time Cleansing Program will help you to cleanse and detoxify your body and reduce your symptoms. You may also choose to use this program to ritualize your moon time and honor the monthly cleansing and revitalizing of your body.

At Ovulation–Use INNER BEAUTY DOUCHE, if necessary, for symptoms of vaginal infection.

About 3 to 7 Days Before Next Menstrual Period–Begin DIURETIC TEA (page 86), one cup per day, to prevent or relieve bloating. Continue until period ends. Begin MOON–TIME TONIC (page 217), two cups per day between meals, to prevent other symptoms of PMS. If symptoms are not controlled with this schedule, experiment with beginning Moon–Time Tonic, one cup per day, a few days earlier in the cycle.

To Relieve Constipation–The last few days before your menstrual period are an excellent time for a professional colonic, preceded by a HOT CASTOR–OIL ABDOMINAL WRAP (page 186) the night before. Or use Hot Castor–Oil Wrap alone the night before your period begins.

First Day of The Menstrual Period–LOWER–BODY LYMPH MASSAGE (page 162) with mustard "HOT FOOT" SOAK (page 162). If necessary, increase MOON–TIME TONIC (page 217) to three cups per day throughout menstrual period.

For Cramps–SOOTHING "HOT SEAT" BATH (page 155) with marjoram, lavender, and/or chamomile essential oils. YOGA ARCH POSE VARIATIONS (page 124). HOT CASTOR–OIL ABDOMINAL WRAP (page 186). Progesterone Cream applied to abdomen (page 142).

For Heavy Flow–SOOTHING "HOT SEAT" BATH (page 155) with geranium, cypress, and/or rose essential oils.

For Breast Tenderness or Mood Swings–Apply progesterone cream or roll–on to skin (follow directions of your health professional).

At End of Menstrual Period–INNER BEAUTY DOUCHE (page 218) to restore acid balance to vagina.

PREPARING FOR A HEALTHY MENOPAUSE

Just as menstruation is often treated as taboo in our culture, menopause is generally considered a time of loss. Other cultures do not necessarily view menopause in this light; many embrace it as a time when women achieve the peak of their power. Indian lore recognizes the power of older women. In many Native American tribes, when women stop menstruating, they are allowed entry into the revered Grandmother Lodge. These elder women are respected for their wisdom, and are believed to have great power because they are holding on to their "wise blood."

A comfortable menopause is simply an outgrowth of a healthy lifestyle. Menopause does not happen all of a sudden, but takes place gradually over time. Most women undergo menopause between the ages of forty and fifty, but the timing is partly determined by how they prepared their bodies in their thirties and even earlier. While there is nothing to dread in the cessation of menses, it can be delayed for many years by following a proper diet, using supplements, promoting proper elimination, and maintaining a positive attitude. The older you are when menopause occurs, the easier it will be.

Many women and men reach the true fullness of their beauty as they age gracefully. The secret lies in maintaining vibrant, radiant health. There is no time in life when following my program will pay off more dramatically than when you are older. The more you have kept your body clean and clear over

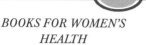
the years, the easier your transition will be.

The popular perception of menopausal women as depressed, irritable and sometimes crazy must be debunked! Menopause is a natural, universal event, not a time of acute crisis. All that happens is, over a period of time, you stop menstruating and can no longer reproduce. In a study of 2,500 middle–aged women by the Women's Research Institute in Massachusets, more than 70% of those experiencing menopause reported neutral or relieved feelings at seeing the last of their periods.

Admittedly, some women do have a difficult time of it. But depression and mood swings may have more to do with our cultural attitudes than with hormonal changes. In Africa and Japan, where aging enhances a woman's status, menopause is viewed as an achievement. Not surprisingly, women in those countries report fewer hot flashes and lower levels of discontent.

Experts are beginning to realize that many of the problems of menopause, the ups and downs and the irritability that accompanies them, may understandably result from a lack of sleep due to hot flashes. Up to 15% of women experience flashes so severe that they are awakened several times during the night. The effects of sleep deprivation are well documented.

Some 70% of menopausal women occasionally experience hot flashes–feelings of extreme heat caused by fluctuating levels of estrogen. They come on unexpectedly and last from one to five minutes. During the "flash", heart rates increase and skin temperatures rise. Afterward, body temperatures fall slightly and one may sweat and feel chilled.

Many menopausal women experience decreased sexual enjoyment. The decline in libido is likely to be related to discomfort resulting from vaginal soreness or dryness, which can be treated with topical lubricants and other natural methods.

There are many books written about menopause and women's health in general. Make it your responsibility to become fully informed! Talking with others who are going through menopause can help make it easier. Finding a doctor who is truly your partner is also very important. You need to be able to have a series of conversations with your doctor, not just a two minute exchange. Many doctors are now introducing the subject to patients and are spending time explaining treatment alternatives.

"ALTERNATIVE" THERAPIES AND ACTIVITIES FOR MENOPAUSE

In addition to following the "Smooth Cycle Checklist" on page 215, try some of these natural remedies.

* Regular sexual activity (including masturbation) helps forestall vaginal dryness and soreness.

* If you experience sexual discomfort, rub your favorite vegetable oil or castor oil on your vaginal area.

* Kegel exercises, done by contracting the muscles you use to stop your flow of urine midstream, can help prevent urinary incontinence. Do 10 repeti-

---

BOOKS FOR WOMEN'S HEALTH

There have been many fantastic books written by women for women. The following are some of my favorites.

Women's Bodies, Women's Wisdom *by Christine Northrup, M.D. (Bantam)*

The New Our Bodies, Our Selves *by Boston's Women's Health Collective (Simon and Schuster)*

Super Nutrition for Women *by Ann Louise Gittleman, M.S. (Pocket)*

Healthy Healing *by Linda Rector Page (Healthy Healing)*

The Pause *by Loni Barbach (Penguin)*

Super Nutrition for Menopause *by Ann Louise Gittleman, M.S. (Pocket)*

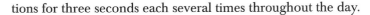

tions for three seconds each several times throughout the day.

* If you do experience a hot flash, please don't fight it. Try to relax until the discomfort eases. Open the windows, lower the thermostat, layer your clothing and try one of the deep breathing activities I describe on pages 135 through 139. Do the Yoga Stress Releaser on page 124. Remember, it is a natural function and will pass soon!

* Stay away from spicy foods and cut back on caffeine and alcohol. These substances will all enhance the hot flashes. Smokers often have more difficulty with menopause.

* Increase your physical activity. Studies show that physically active women experience half as many hot flashes as women who do not work out.

* Follow the supplement regime I describe on page 72. Vitamin E may reduce hot flashes enormously and relieve vaginal dryness. It may also reduce the risk of heart disease and cancer. In addition to B–complex vitamins, women should be careful to get plenty of calcium–rich foods and calcium–magnesium supplements to guard against osteoporosis in later years, which so often occurs as the hormone balance changes after menopause. Stress also depletes calcium. Women should also not overdo their protein consumption, because protein can remove calcium from the bones.

* In addition, take 500 mg. of Evening Primrose Oil capsules four times daily.

* Take Royal Jelly daily (page 206).

* Plant estrogens, found in soybean products such as tofu, are thought to mimic the effects of estrogen and so may help alleviate vaginal dryness and hot flashes. The recipes containing tofu on pages 104 through 105 will be beneficial to incorporate into your diet on a regular basis. In addition, there are many herbal products specifically designed to assist in balancing your hormones. Herbs specifically beneficial for menopause include Dong Quai, Red Raspberry, Licorice Root, Black Cohosh and Wild Yam. You may check in your local health–food store for specific combination products appropriate for your symptoms.

As never before, our fellow humans and our overburdened planet need the guidance of healthy, emotionally centered, and spiritually mature "elders". Choose now to take your rightful place among those who will show a better way for future generations. Keep your mind and body clean and clear, and bring the world along with you.

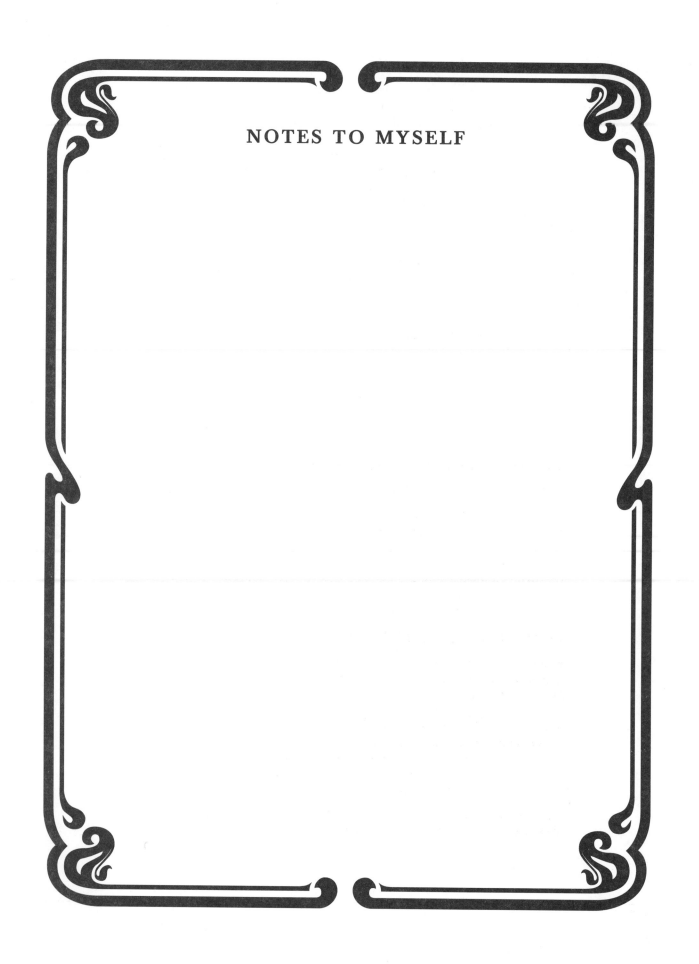

NOTES TO MYSELF

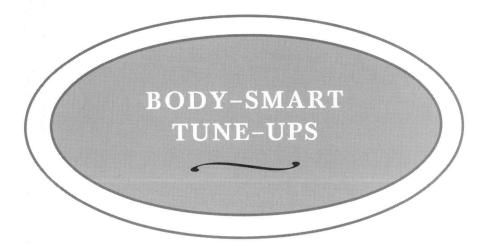

BODY-SMART TUNE-UPS:
ONE, THREE & EIGHT DAY PLANS

Now that you have finished the 21–Day Program, I am sure you want to know how you can incorporate what you have learned into the rest of your life. Try to develop the habit of lightening your diet and cleansing your body and mind on a regular basis. Many of my clients go on a seasonal cleansing regimen as a means of rejuvenation. Find the cycle that works best for you. Make a commitment to repeat the 21–Day Program twice a year—spring and fall are the traditional times for cleansing.

REJUVENATION TOUCH-UPS

Keep in mind that you should undertake the Rejuvenation Touch–up Programs only if you have been following the principles of the Clean and Clear Diet on a regular basis. If you have been eating all sorts of foods, improperly combined, you must prepare your body before you jump into anything too strenuous. I must emphasize that the Rejuvenation Touch–up Programs are not crash diets. The more that you do the entire cleansing program, not just change the way you eat, the more physical and mental benefits you will derive.

Experiment with the rejuvenating possibilities offered by these periodic cleansing programs to discover which ones are right for your needs. As always, be easy on yourself and just do the best you can do. You will achieve results even if you don't do it perfectly.

ONE–DAY LIQUID CLEANSING DIET

I recommend that you rest and cleanse your system one day each week with the One–Day Liquid Cleansing Diet. This lifelong rejuvenation strategy is an effective tool for managing your weight and for cellulite control. The day you set aside for this diet is also an excellent time to receive a professional massage, since you are resting your digestive system and releasing toxins and tension. I like to do this diet regularly on Mondays. If I have wavered from the Clean and Clear Diet over the weekend, a Monday cleansing is a great way to begin the week with new energy and inspiration.

BREAKFAST: LIVER FLUSH #1 OR #2 (pages 85 to 86).

MIDMORNING SNACK: Optional–Fruit juice of choice, freshly squeezed (if you need the extra energy boost).

LUNCH: PROTEIN DRINK of choice (pages 107 to 110).

MIDAFTERNOON SNACK: CLEANSING JUICE BLEND of choice (page 110). Drink one cup of DIURETIC TEA (page 86) one hour before dinner.

DINNER: POTASSIUM BROTH or VEGETABLE BISQUE of choice (pages 92 to 97).

THROUGHOUT THE DAY: Drink HERBAL PURIFICATION TEA (page 84) between meals.

THREE–DAY REJUVENATION INTENSIVE

The Three–Day Rejuvenation Intensive is a wonderful way to prepare for a special event, or to lighten up your body and your mind. If you feel yourself coming down with a cold or the flu, this Three–Day Intensive is also a good way to give your digestive system a rest so that your body can direct its energies toward healing.

Day 1

ON AWAKENING: One 8–ounce glass of HOT LEMON–WATER FLUSH (page 80). Prepare HERBAL PURIFICATION TEA (page 84) for the day; drink it throughout the day between meals. Use INSPIROL (cleansing inhalant) (page 135).

MORNING CLEANSING: DRY BRUSH MASSAGE (page 144). Follow with a hot shower, finishing with a one–minute cold splash.

BREAKFAST: PAPAYA COMPLEXION BREAKFAST (page 90).

LUNCH: CARROT SHAKE (page 110), as much as you want.

MIDAFTERNOON SNACK: Vegetable juice of choice.

DINNER: SUPER SALAD with sunflower seeds (page 98) and FAT-LOSS DRESSING of choice (pages 100 to 101); POTASSIUM BROTH (page 92), one cup.

EXERCISE: OXYGENATION COCKTAIL (page 82). Follow with YOGA STRESS RELEASERS (page 124). If you are feeling well, enjoy thirty minutes of brisk walking.

EVENING ACTIVITY: "HOT FOOT" SOAK (page 162), followed by professional massage.

Day 2

ON AWAKENING: Drink one glass of HYDRATING DRINK (page 81). Prepare HERBAL PURIFICATION TEA (page 84) for the day; drink it throughout the day between meals. Use INSPIROL (cleansing inhalant) (page 135).

MORNING CLEANSING: DRY BRUSH MASSAGE (page 144), followed by ALTERNATING HOT AND COLD SHOWER, ending with cold.

BREAKFAST: LIVER FLUSH #1 (page 85).

LUNCH: TAHINI SHAKE (page 110), as much as you want.

MIDAFTERNOON SNACK: Vegetable juice of choice.

DINNER: HIJIKI STIR-FRY (page 106), with one cup of POTASSIUM BROTH (page 92).

EXERCISE: OXYGENATION COCKTAIL (page 82) followed by ANTI-GRAVITY TONE-UP (page 122) and ANTIGRAVITY FACIAL MASSAGE (page 174). If you are feeling well, enjoy brisk walking for thirty minutes.

EVENING ACTIVITY: TUMMY MASSAGE (page 187), followed by HOT CASTOR-OIL ABDOMINAL WRAP (page 186).While Castor-Oil Wrap is on, do THREE-PART BREATHING (page 137) and COMPLETE BREATH (page 138). EPSOM SALTS SOAK (page 153), with one tablespoon of baking soda added.

Day 3

ON AWAKENING: Drink one glass of HYDRATING DRINK (page 81). Prepare HERBAL PURIFICATION TEA (page 84) for the day; drink it throughout the day between meals. Use INSPIROL (cleansing inhalant) (page 135).

MORNING CLEANSING: MORNING COLD SPLASH AND RUB (page

xxx), followed by DRY BRUSH MASSAGE (page 144).

Breakfast: LIVER FLUSH #2 (page 86).

Lunch: MAPLE–NUT SHAKE (page 109), as much as you want.

Midafternoon Snack: Vegetable juice of choice.

Dinner: VEGETABLE BISQUE of choice (pages 92 to 97), as much as you want; small SUPER SALAD (page 98).

Exercise: OXYGENATION COCKTAIL (page 82). Follow with YOGA REJUVENATION POSTURES (page 129). If you are feeling well, enjoy brisk walking for thirty minutes.

Evening Activity: Professional colonic, followed by TRANQUILITY BATH (page 156).

EIGHT–DAY SHAPE–UP

To prepare for a special event, when you want to look and feel your best and radiate vitality, follow this eight–day program. If you do not have the time to do the entire 21–Day Program, this intensive Shape–up is excellent for seasonal cleansing, for after the holidays or an overindulgent vacation, for recovering from a major stress, or for any time you want to devote a special eight days to taking care of yourself. To avoid cleansing reactions, please do not begin this program unless you have been on the Clean and Clear Diet for at least one week. Return to the Clean and Clear Diet afterward, and you will continue to enjoy the physical and mental benefits.

Your meals and beverages during the Eight–Day Shape–up are based on the intensive cleansing portion of the 21–Day Program. You begin with the raw–foods portion of this cleansing regimen, and return gently to fruits and raw and cooked vegetables after a two–day liquid fast. The evening activities are an intensified and accelerated version of the cleansing and stress-releasing activities used during the 21–Day Program.

To do the Eight–Day Shape–up, follow all the day–by–day instructions for Day 10 through Day 17, and add the special activities indicated below.

1.   HOT CASTOR–OIL ABDOMINAL WRAP (page 186) every night if possible. Be sure to include the Castor Oil Wrap the nights before your colon cleansings.

2.   Two yoga sessions: DIGESTION TONING POSTURES (page 128) and YOGA REJUVENATION POSTURES (page 129).

3.   UPPER– and LOWER–BODY LYMPH MASSAGE (pages 162 to 163), preceded by "HOT FOOT" SOAK (page 169).

4.   Three breathing–exercises sessions: Each time include THREE–PART

BREATHING (page 137), COMPLETE BREATH (page 138), ALTER-NATE–HEMISPHERE BREATHING (page 139), and BALLOON BREATHING (page 135).

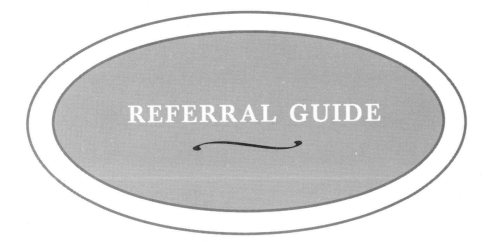

REFERRAL GUIDE

*H*OLISTIC *H*EALTH
*P*RACTITIONERS

*I*f you have decided to seek professional help and cannot find a practitioner near you, contact one of the following organizations. They will refer you to a qualified practitioner in your area.

AMERICAN HOLISTIC MEDICAL ASSOCIATION

4101 Lake Boone Trail #201

Raleigh, N.C. 27607

(919) 787-5181

AMERICAN COLLEGE OF ADVANCEMENT IN MEDICINE

23121 Verdugo Drive #204

Laguna Hills, CA 92653

(800) 532-3688

AMERICAN ASSOCIATION OF NATUROPATHIC PHYSICIANS

2366 Eastlake Avenue E #322

Seattle, WA 98102

(206) 323-7610

AMERICAN ASSOCIATION OF ACUPUNCTURE AND ORIENTAL MEDICINE

433 Front Street

Catasauqua, PA 18032

(610) 433-2448

AMERICAN MASSAGE THERAPY ASSOCIATION

820 Davis Street #100

Evanston, ILL 60201

(312) 761-2682

INTERNATIONAL ASSOCIATION OF COLON THERAPISTS

2051 Hilltop Drive #A11

Redding, CA 96002

(916) 222-1498

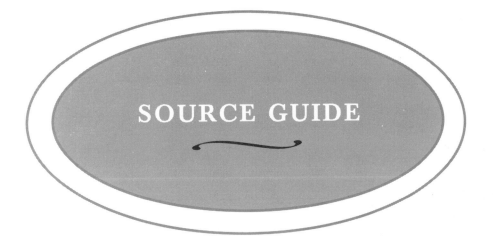

SOURCE GUIDE

I have designed Body–Smart Products especially for those of you who do not have a health-food store near your home or would like to shop by mail!

The products I recommend throughout The Body–Smart System come from an advanced class of integrated state–of–the–art nutrients designed to help you enhance your health by boosting your natural processes and internally cleansing the body of inner toxic pollution. Scientific discoveries have contributed more in the last 10 years than in any preceding time about how nutrition contributes to optimal health; nutritional experts have integrated these highly advanced discoveries in the many natural formulas available today in the natural foods industry.

I make the best of these high quality products available through The Body–Smart Products Catalog.

I have created The Body–Smart Product Kits which allow you to follow the 21-Day Cleansing and Rejuvenation Program and, if you wish, to individualize the Program based on your goals and health history. They are an assortment of products designed to deal with problems such as irregularity, indigestion, weight loss, cellulite, skin problems, stress, PMS, and menopause. The Body–Smart Kits include simple teas, herbal and nutritional supplements, and natural seaweed and aromatherapy products for your skin and bath.

For information on how to order these products and/or about Inner Beauty Retreats, please mail the following request form to:

Body–Smart
3A Gate Five Road
Sausalito, CA   94965

Please send me more information on Body–Smart Products.

NAME _____

ADDRESS _____

_____

TELEPHONE NUMBER_____

☐   *Yes! I would also like information on Inner Beauty Retreats.*

INDEX

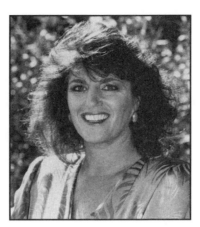

About The Author

Helene Silver has been an educator, nutritionist, and health professional for more than twenty years. She received her educational training at UCLA and taught in the Oakland Public Schools from 1968 to 1976. While teaching school, she studied health and nutrition at The University of California at Berkeley and Antioch University. In 1978 Ms. Silver received a grant from the California Department of Education to develop nutrition education training programs for students, faculty, and food service personnel. She has lectured at the American Association of University Women, the Continuing Education Program for Nurses, the Health Task Force for the Democratic Central Committee, Women Entrepreneurs, and B'nai Brith Women.

In 1980, Ms. Silver founded The Inner Beauty Institute of Sausalito. The Institute specializes in the development of wellness programs tailored to suit personal health concerns. This individualized approach focuses on detoxifying, rejuvenating, and revitalizing the body. The Institute uses colonic irrigations, full-body scrubs, lymphatic massage, and herbal steam baths, accompanied by nutritional and stress reduction counseling

Ms. Silver also conducts seven–day health retreats throughout the year at select locations in Northern California. Her clients participate in rejuvenation programs with special emphasis on bodywork, stress reduction techniques, mountain hikes, and individualized cleansing and weight–loss diets.